Acknowledgements

I want to thank all those who contributed to the stories acknowledged in this book.

Alzheimer's is a disease causing the mind to become twisted and distorted, sometimes to a degree of becoming violent. Dementia is another form causing the mind to become twisted and distorted. Those suffering from the effects of these mind tangling problems often wander away and become lost in reality. It is the debilitating effects of this horrible disease into the depths of the normal brain that cause the normal to revert to the abnormal. Thanks to those who have helped contribute. These stories are not meant to be disrespectful, but to help you find humor or help understand the invasions that can destroy our once healthy brains. It can happen to you!

My mother suffered from Dementia brought on from stress. In January 2000 my sister, Carol, was brutally murdered at the hands of her foster child. Mother could not face this horrible tragedy. That same year a child Mother raised had a massive heart attack at the young age of 47, and that same year her last sister out of a family of 16 children died. In November the same year, we lost my step dad to a massive heart attack. The doctor explained she reverted into a form of Dementia to keep from having a mental breakdown. She became my child, I became her mother. She was quick to tell you, in a heartbeat, that she had some things "tucked" away in the back of her brain and she was not ready to go there. This book was written from a diary I kept during those years and out of love and respect for my precious mother. It was not easy to break through some of the barriers that surrounded the problem, but it did make me realize the importance of trying to help others understand this strange unwanted disease of the mind.

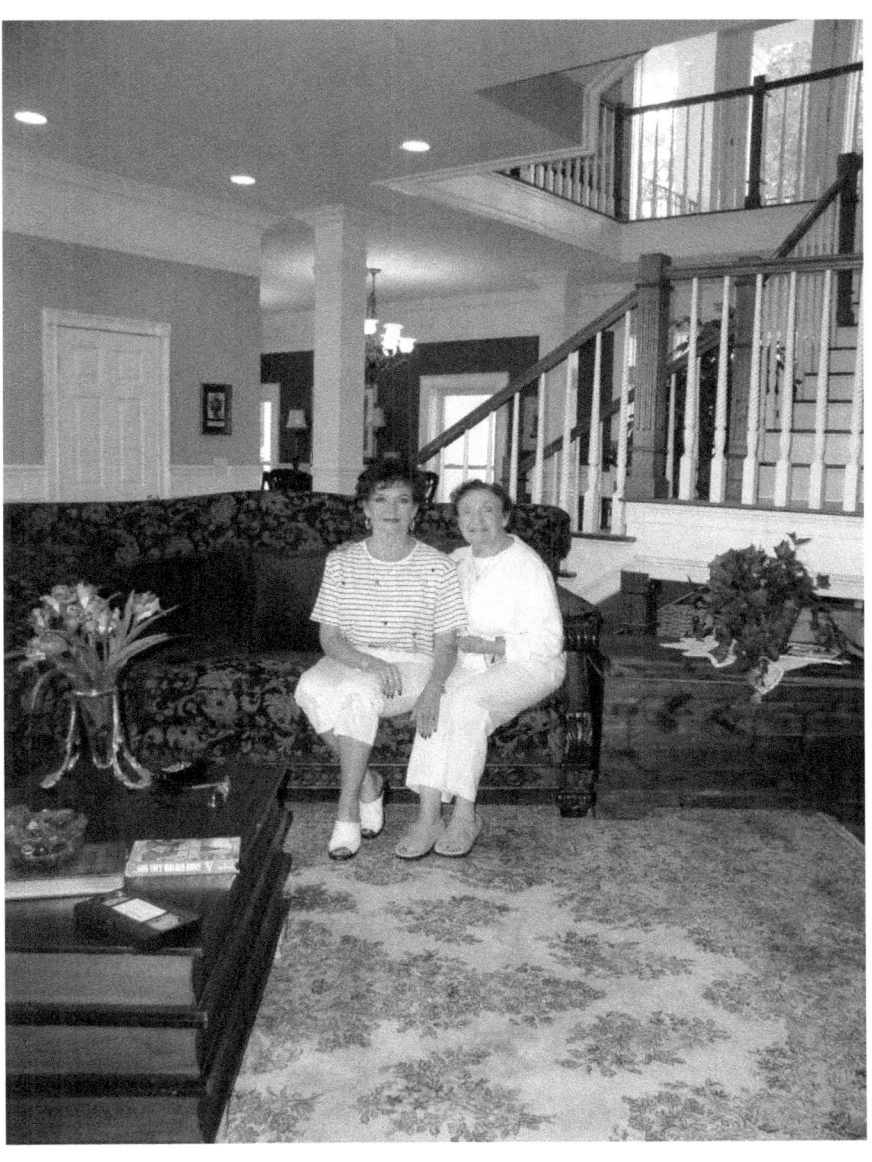

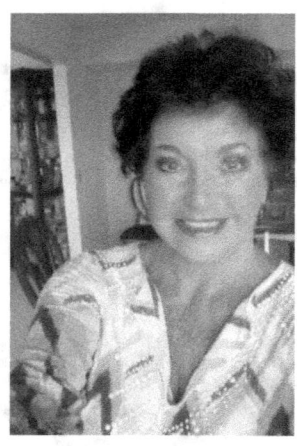

Author

Editor: Kenneth D. Wilson

Other Books:

- *In the Sweet By and By*

- *Take A Walk Through Life With LED Light*

- *A True Story*

DEDICATION

I dedicate this book to all caregivers caring for someone with memory loss. May you enjoy these heartfelt stories and may they help give you strength to endure. May they linger in your mind knowing that you too may become the victim of a perplexing disease yet to be stopped and often misunderstood? Hopefully, if this happens, you will have that special person caring for you. We give back to those who have given to us. It is our parents, for without them, we would not be here.

I also give a special dedication to my daughter, Kimberly Ann Hunt Verge and granddaughter, Christie, for their love and devotion to me, and for the time they gave to their grandmother, Emily.

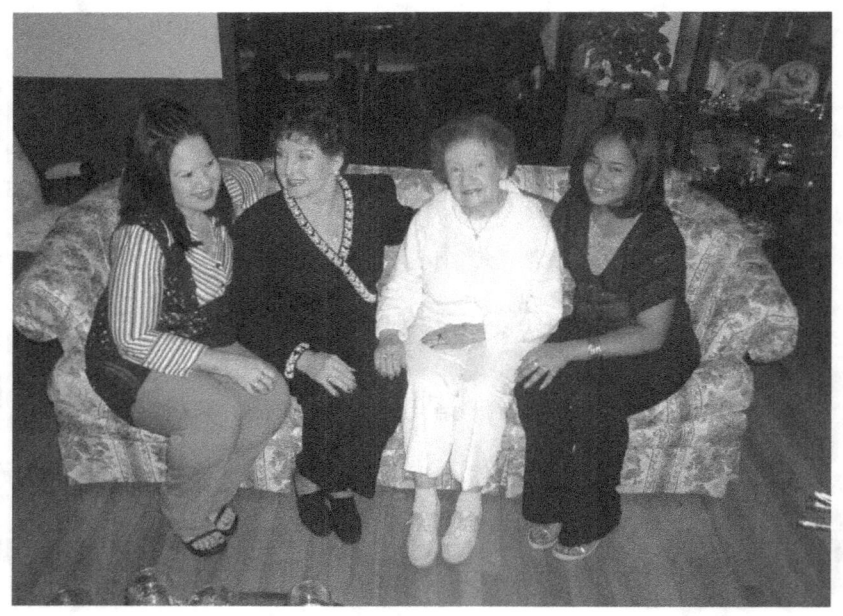

Kim, Joyce, Mother and Christie (Christmas 2006 – Emily 87 years old)

INDEX OF A TWISTED MIND

INTRODUCTION

Many have wondered why I wrote this book, but it was because as I walked through the ten years of mother's plight with dementia, I felt I became very knowledgeable about this disease. It is a disease that any of us could face one day and to know and understand some of the signs and symptoms could help in diagnosing this problem. It is a disease that does not differentiate age. In the UK alone, there is over 17,000 young people with dementia, no doubt an underestimate.

Alzheimer's is a form of dementia; however, there are many forms of dementia. Often the younger get Alzheimer's, and older get dementia going into Alzheimer's.

CHAPTER 1 – Symptoms of Dementia

It was Friday at the HairPort & Wellness Center in Jasper, AL. The four of us sat at the fifteen foot manicure table. A table that had held many clients over the past twenty-seven years and could tell a lot of stories if it could talk. It was the end of a hard week. We finally rested our feet and sat discussing our association with someone close to us having Alzheimer's or Dementia. Dana, who had served as manager for over ten years, began telling a first story about her grandmother diagnosed with Alzheimer's. She was caregiver to her granny, who still lived alone; however, one night her granny called needing milk. Her story brought about our first round of hysterical laughter. Dana recalled Ron, her husband, offered to take the milk to "Little Granny." When he knocked on the door, Little Granny opened the door, stark naked, as if nothing was out of order. "Oh, she did have socks on," piped in Dana as we all started to roll with laughter. Ron quickly threw his arm up over his face to shield the view, reached out and handed Little Granny the milk and proceeded to leave. She quickly said, "Wait a minute Ron, I have to give you some change." We could not help but scream with laughter as we sat visualizing his dilemma and with that each began telling their tales of the "Twisted Mind."

As you read through these true tales, it may ring a bell to someone you know going through this strange disease of the mind. May the following simple hints help recognize problems.

1. **Does the loved one forget your name or who you are?**

2. **Can the loved one make decisions when and how to bath?**

3. **Can the loved one drive or have problems trying to cook?**

4. **Can the loved one handle banking and bill paying?**

5. Does the loved one tell the same story, word for word, over and over again or talk about visiting someone long passed?

6. Does the loved one hide things or get agitated easy?

7. Does the loved one feel scared and often think someone is trying to harm them?

If your loved one has these problems, seek professional help.

Taken from the "Alzheimer's Disease" Web Site.

Every person is unique and dementia affects people differently - no two people will have symptoms that develop in exactly the same way. An individual's personality, general health and social situation are all important factors in determining the impact of dementia on him or her.

The most common early symptoms of dementia are:

MEMORY LOSS

Declining memory, especially short-term memory, is the most common early symptom of dementia. People with ordinary forgetfulness can still remember other facts associated with the thing they have forgotten. For example they may briefly forget their next-door neighbour's name but they still know the person they are talking to is their next-door neighbour. A person with dementia will not only forget their neighbor's name but also the context.

DIFFICULTY PERFORMING FAMILIAR TASKS

People with dementia often find it hard to complete everyday tasks that are so familiar we usually do not think about how to do them. A person with dementia may not know in what order to put clothes on or the steps for preparing a meal.

PROBLEMS WITH LANGUAGE

Occasionally everyone has trouble finding the right word but a person with dementia often forgets simple words or substitute's unusual words, making speech or writing hard to understand.

DISORIENTATION TO TIME AND PLACE

We sometimes forget the day of the week or where we are going but people with dementia can become lost in familiar places such as the road they live in, forget where they are or how they got there, and not know how to get back home. A person with dementia may also confuse night and day.

POOR OR DECREASED JUDGEMENT

People with dementia may dress inappropriately, wearing several layers of clothes on a warm day or very few on a cold day.

PROBLEMS WITH KEEPING TRACK OF THINGS

A person with dementia may find it difficult to follow a conversation or keep up with paying their bills.

MISPLACING THINGS

Anyone can temporarily misplace his or her wallet or keys. A person with dementia may put things in unusual places such as an iron in the fridge or a wristwatch in the sugar bowl.

CHANGES IN MOOD OR BEHAVIOUR

Everyone can become sad or moody from time to time. A person with dementia may become unusually emotional and experience rapid mood swings for no apparent reason. Alternatively a person with dementia may show less emotion than was usual previously.

CHANGES IN PERSONALITY

A person with dementia may seem different from his or her usual self in ways that are difficult to pinpoint. A person may become suspicious, irritable, depressed, apathetic or anxious and agitated especially in situations where memory problems are causing difficulties.

LOSS OF INITIATIVE

At times everyone can become tired of housework, business activities, or social obligations. However a person with dementia may become very passive, sitting in front of the television for hours, sleeping more than usual, or appear to lose interest in hobbies.

If you are experiencing any of these symptoms or are concerned about a friend or relative, visit your doctor and discuss your concerns.

Unfortunately, this dreaded disease can shorten one's life span; however, it has been known that some forms of Alzheimer's victims can live for years. A simple one minute test can often identify those at risk. This valuable information came from the "Prevention.Com." web site: How many animals can you name in a minute? It's a fun keep-the-kids-occupied-in-the-car game, but when UK scientists asked 136 volunteers to play, they found a way to detect early-stage dementia. People with early Alzheimer's named an average of 10 to 15 animals or fruits within the time allowed. Healthy adults, however, listed 20 to 25. While the Alzheimer's group thought of everyday words such as cat and apple, they left out others that aren't used as often, such as zebra and kiwi. The pattern was so consistent that researchers correctly identified ill patients based solely on word lists. The potential payoff: Early detection may someday give scientists a better shot at slowing disease progression.

The 10 Absolutes of Care giving for Alzheimer's Patients: Never ARGUE, instead, AGREE. Never REASON, instead, DIVERT. Never

SHAME, instead, DISTRACT. Never LECTURE, instead, REASSURE. Never "REMEMBER," instead, REMINISCE. Never "I TOLD YOU," instead, REPEAT. Never "YOU CANT," instead, "do WHAT YOU CAN." Never COMMAND OR DEMAND, instead ASK OR MODEL. Never CONDESCEND, instead, ENCOURAGE OR PRAISE. Never FORCE, instead, REINFORCE.

The following problems were taken from The Alzheimer's Foundation Web site:

- Trouble with new memories
- Relying on memory helpers
- Trouble finding words
- Struggling to complete familiar actions
- Confusion about time, place or people
- Misplacing familiar objects
- Onset of new depression or irritability
- Making bad decisions
- Personality changes
- Loss of interest in important responsibilities
- Seeing or hearing things

- Expressing false beliefs

Now that you have experienced a little insight to problems that develop with memory loss, let us give you some uplifting views of what goes on inside the "Twisted Mind" from those suffering with this unfortunate disease. I am sure if you have an association with one with this problem, you too could add some additional interesting stories.

This book was written with love and respect to those going through memory loss from Alzheimer's or Dementia. It was also written for those going through the role as caregiver and hoping in some small way it will bring an insight to the other side of the disease. Being caregiver to my mother for several years, I began seeing her little twisted mind unraveling, making drastic turns and watching her 87 years of life revert back to that of a child. I often found her in my clothes with the pants rolled up, wearing my rings, sweeping the walkways to our home in my fancy jackets and closing doors shutting out the "unwelcome." She would often put chairs up against the front door for safety, listened for the unknown and wondered through the house looking for a "pee pot." She was born in the heart of the Appalachian Mountains of Kentucky into poverty. She lived in a house high on the mountains away from flood waters and without indoor facilities. She kept her shoes off the floor to prevent rats from carrying them off. She hid her precious things from those who might take a "lik'n to them. She was the first born daughter to a mother who birthed sixteen children. She would be the last of the "litter" and never hesitated to fight for her rights. A tough 4'11" woman and a handful to care for, with a heart full of love gave me the strength to endure the ravages of a disease still hard to understand. Yes, I went to bed exhausted, my nerves were often shot, I began to suffer with high blood pressure and I wondered what tomorrow would bring. When I looked at her sweet face, the problems seemed to melt away.

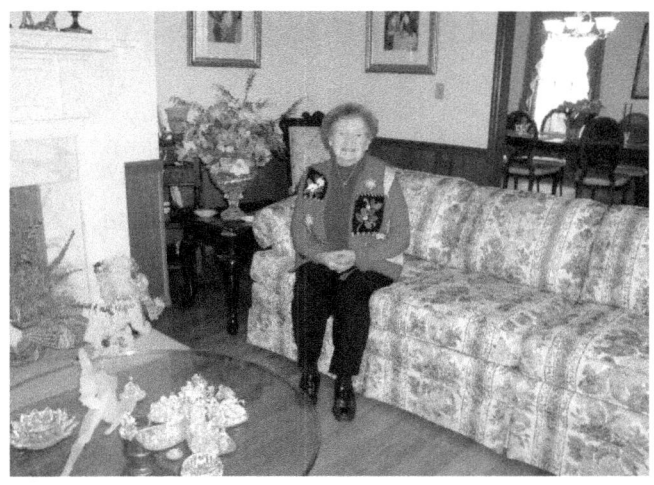

Mother loved Christmas, opening gifts. She especially enjoyed the cakes, pies and goodies.   She also loved looking pretty. Her sweater was a special gift from Phyllis, her best friend.   Christmas 2006

CHAPTER 2 – A Lost Day

I first noticed serious changes in my mother when Carol was taken away from us at the hands of her foster child. She was the youngest of three girls, Shirley, Joyce and Carol. The doctor said mother put everything into the back of her mind to keep from going insane. She was unable to cope with the devastating losses she would endure that harsh year. Carol was murdered January 17, 2000;, the same year, Curtis, the child of her brother she had raised after the deaths of his parents, would die of a massive heart attack; her last sister, Ruby would die in October; and then lastly my stepfather died suddenly the day after Thanksgiving while she made coffee, leaving her now twice a widow. It was a trying and horrifying year, but what would come next was a different form of death. It was the death of the brain, twisting her mind and changing my mother forever. At first, it nearly broke my heart, but as I continued my new role as caregiver, it became a challenge to try different methods to understand how to help give mother quality life. At the same time, I worked on my own stress level knowing I had to have the patience of "Jobe." Mother reverted back to childhood that year and I reverted from daughter to mother that same year. Both our lives changed forever during that horrible year. It was like a nightmare. I felt our family had been marked by death.

Days became nonexistent to mother. She lived for the moment. Christmas no longer had meaning, or Thanksgiving, Mother's Day or any given special day of the year. She opened a gift with enthusiasm, hid her new treasures and soon forgot the occasion. Her birthday remained in her mind for a few moments, not minutes, moments, but she also had now lost the days of the week, and months of the year. She could no longer remember the year, day or time as witnessed by an alarm clock that sat silent on her nightstand. Her life no longer had meaning. She no longer had goals, wrote letters, or sent special cards a trait for which she was known. She no longer had grocery lists on the refrigerator, made her famous buttermilk biscuits or washed and ironed clothes. She no longer drove the car, but could convince a stranger that she still had her license and drove when she had "a mind for." She could make you look bad in front of the doctor if she complained not wanting to go to her appointment. She would whisper to those around her that I did not know what I was talking about. At first my feelings were bruised often, but as I worked with Mother I realized I would have to make the changes within myself and accept her unhealthy thinking. The doctor might ask, "Mrs. Smith do you still drive?" If Mother said yes, I would intervene and explain that she does not drive anymore. I realized this was an embarrassment to mother, causing frustration and anger and decided to take a different approach. I began getting behind mother at the doctor when questions were directed to mother, and shake my head yes or no behind mother's back.

You may ask yourself this question. How do you become a caregiver? It is a new job with a new title, very stressful and without experience. It is not awarded to you, but handed down when no one else chooses to accept the position. I noticed little things that grew into major things the early part of the year Carol passed. When I made my usual calls home, I often asked, "Mom, what did you cook for dinner?" She paused and I could hear her ask Dad, "Frank, honey, what did we have for dinner?" From there it became more serious, hiding her purse and taking hours to find it. She also began accusing others of taking her things, blocking the doors with chairs, trying to cook and having difficulty making biscuits or placing plastic containers of food in a hot oven. When she could not remember how to make biscuits, I knew something unnatural was happening. She hid candy saying the children would eat it so she put it away for safe keeping. It was the little things I began noticing, nothing serious, but then as time progressed it became more difficult to reason with her. Small things became big things and then the confrontations followed. I remember during those first months she actually got so angry she slapped me and spit in my face. It hurt my feelings more than causing pain from the blow. This was not my mother, I thought, but someone taking over her mind and body. She soon progressed to no longer cooking, but thinking she cooked; not cleaning the bathrooms, but thinking she cleaned, and finally trying to convince me she had bathed, when I knew she had not bathed. When it became evident she had serious memory problems, I began playing mind games using reverse psychology. Sometimes it worked, sometimes it didn't. It saved the knock down drag out verbal fights that left us both totally exhausted. At the beginning it was easier to get baths over with in the evenings. I used the term, "Mom, let's get our baths and curl our hair so we can get up early and go shopping." It was a magical word to her twisted little mind. Later, this reversed to morning baths. Demanding caused friction, but giving her a reason created positive results. I no longer argued when insisting she had mopped, cleaned, swept and did all the laundry while I worked. When she smiled, I agreed that the house looked beautiful and I was proud she kept it that way. She would meet me at the door, wearing whatever she found in my closet, explaining how tired she was from her day of work. I had realized it was easier for me to make changes. Her mind had already made them for her. I did find things she could still do. I did the laundry while she did the dishes, but of course, I had to prepare the dishwater. She would rinse her dishes, but use no soap if I did not make the dishwater for her. It gave her a job rather than to run the dishwasher. After all, she did a great job washing those dishes and it was something she could still do. Dishwashing by hand was part of her past, not present. She would still put her shoes in a chair at night from the "rats."

Sunday mornings gave me some time while mother slept, to check my emails and start breakfast.   I cooked breakfast every morning. Once on a cold day and I decided to serve breakfast in front of the fireplace while watching the news. Mom seemed to be sleeping longer hours and on this particular morning I wondered how long she would sleep. Sometimes I took a peak into her room to make sure she was alright as her congestive heart failure kept me attentive to her needs. She finally came out of her bedroom, but seemed to be in a quiet mood that particular morning as she ate.

After breakfast, I did the laundry, leaving her two girdles hanging on the washer lid to air dry as I planned later to do a little Christmas and grocery shopping. The last of the laundry was finally drying in the dryer and I ironed the pillow cases to put back on the beds. Suddenly I noticed mom's underwear was no longer on the washer lid air drying. I began hunting, first looking in her chest drawers, then in mine and last in the guest bedroom drawers. I could not believe how "quick" she was, not to mention how quiet while she gathered these personal items that belonged to her. No girdles. I searched the house finally looking in the garbage. They were nowhere to be found. I asked her where she put her girdles and she replied, "Well, Joyce Ann I haven't seen them." (She called me Joyce Ann when she was annoyed with me.) "How would I know?" Of course, how would she know? The mind is twisted and the thought was gone. Oh well, I thought, I will add them to the list with the missing velour top that never emerged earlier in the week. Where the darned girdles could be hidden definitely was a new mystery. The house was only so big and there were only so many places to "tuck" things away. Thinking I overlooked the girdles, I began searching all over again. It was like her "lost day," and the girdles were gone. Finally I tired, gave up and we left to go shopping. How could girdles just disappear? It could drive you crazy, I thought as we drove away from the house.

I glanced over watching her sweet, innocent face, knowing she could not tell me where those stupid girdles had been hidden. She rode along, happy and content as she sang, "Jingle Bells." I often wondered how one person could find such great hiding places. When I played hide-and-go-seek as a child, I found wonderful places to hide, but never good enough not to be found. Here I am an adult and I could not find girdles, socks, tops, purses, candy, cookies and pots and pans. The list grew daily, not to mention keys and sometimes my cell phone.

When mom lived in her apartment I continued to buy socks thinking she did not have enough. Christmas, Mother's Day and

Birthday I would add beautiful colored socks to match her outfits to the list of gifts. I often hunted for matching socks for her clothes, but often giving up without finding a good match and settling for a neutral color. When I moved mother out of her apartment I found socks stashed everywhere even in the kitchen drawers. Now she had a complete drawer full of socks of every color, probably 75 pairs of socks or possibly more! It was the same with underwear except I still could not find those girdles. Same with bras, but she did have a wonderful assortment of socks, handkerchiefs, bras, panties and girdles. My thoughts still raced wondering where she could have hidden those two girdles that had been air drying on the washer lid. Sometimes I wondered if I was losing it. I dumped these items from my gift lists as I knew they would someday show up in a strange place. Sometimes I would turn and ask, "Mom, you want an ice-cream?" It was a treat she gave us as a child, now she was the child and the favor was returned.

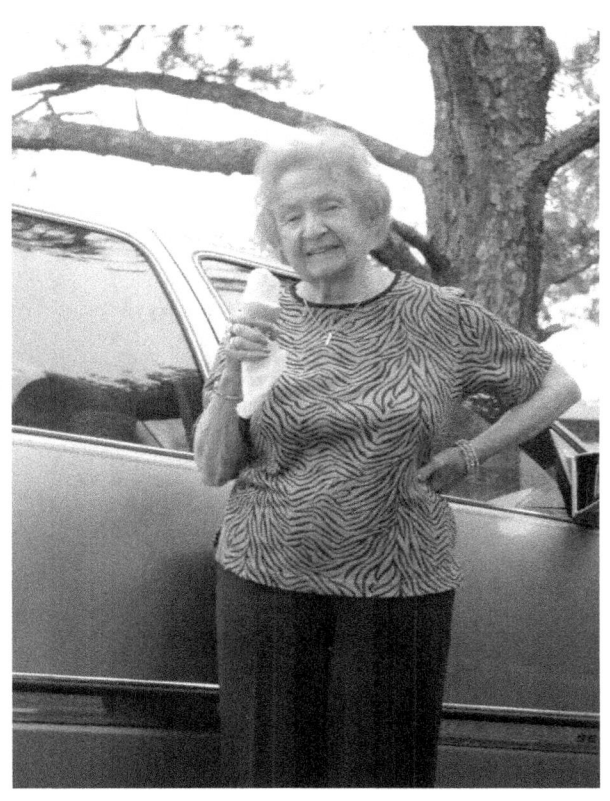

Mother enjoying a favorite treat.

CHAPTER 3 – Pistol Pack n' Momma

Spring was an exciting time for Ms. Emily. She had never lived in an apartment, but now that Dad was gone, I had to sell her house and move her to Alabama near me. There was no one left in Harlan, KY to care for her. The mountains had been her life with neighbors a "stone's throw away." The complex I chose was for elderly people, no pets and no children. The apartment I chose had three bedrooms, eat-in kitchen with bay window, two and one half baths with large vanities for her to primp, combination living room, dining room, and study with beautiful bookcases and built in stereo system. It also had a large finished attic and a car port in the back which made a perfect spot for a covered swing. She had her own private patio with a fenced in yard for flower beds. It was the most desirable of all the units in the complex and I felt lucky to get such a special place. With no children or pets the atmosphere was warm, cozy and safe. In the center of the complex was a small wash room storing brooms for sweeping. The walk ways inside the courtyard were covered and Ms. Emily loved sweeping and kept all the walk ways clean, even during bad weather. Everyone teased about her sweeping and sometimes a neighbor got in on the action with their broom and joined in. One stray leaf blown back on that walk way never stayed long when mother was around.

My salon and wellness center was no more than one mile away making it convenient to check on mother daily. Through the salon, I was introduced to Phyllis by her daughter Yolanda. Being recently divorced, Phyllis needed something to do. It was a happy day for both me and mother. I called several times each day, but also paid Phyllis to take mother on outings four days a week. It was on one off days for Phyllis that I could not get mother to answer her phone. Being a worrier, I left my client with wet hair sitting in my chair, climbed into the car and drove to the complex. Immediately I saw mother with her broom just outside her apartment door talking to a neighbor. As I got closer to mother I noticed a big "bulge" in her right pants pocket. I reached down and patted her pocket and said, "What in the world do you have in your pocket?" She looked kind of funny, turned a little pale and mumbled, "Nothing." I realized she had her 38 Smith and Wesson snub nosed revolver in her pocket and pulled it out. The neighbor looked extremely shocked and I proceeded to tell her that she could not carry a gun without a permit. That did not faze her. She became angry and said, "Oh Joyce Ann, everyone carries a gun. Why your dad always carried his gun every day. I have to protect myself when I am outside. Someone might try to hurt me." The neighbor just stood there and listened. I said, "Well, mother I will put your gun up so no one will get it." With that I walked inside her apartment, hid the gun for retrieval later and went back to work. I had taken the bullets out long ago, but the poor neighbor did not know mother had an empty gun in her pocket. I thought back and laughed thinking how scared the lady probably was realizing she had been talking to my mother at near "gunpoint." When I returned to my salon I announced that Ms. Emily was sweeping the walkways and carrying her .38 for protection. Everyone roared with laughter. It was funny, but it was also nerve wracking. Our family was gun lovers, mother's father had been a gunsmith and my father had been a police officer. We always carried guns in the mountains, but in the city, it was different. You had to have a permit. That was the day I began to realize the seriousness of mother's illness. I later sneaked the gun out and never allowed her to have it again. She missed it for only a very short time, but soon the gun was like the girdles. If it was out of sight, it was out of mind.

After the gun incident I began finding knives under her pillow, screwdrivers or scissors for "protection" at night in her night stand beside her bed. She began putting brooms by her bed or the yard rake. She always propped chairs up against her doors for security. If she slept late, I became scared that something was wrong. It was almost impossible to get into her door for the chairs, stools or whatever she could stack against the doors at night. The apartment had dead bolt locks, but she could not understand that she was safe inside. I could see the paranoia getting worse, not to mention that evenings brought on confusion.

I soon realized mother was having "sun downing syndrome." If I took her to my home for dinner she would say, "It's getting late and my family will be worried." I would say, "What family mother?" She would say, "Oh mom and dad and Woodrow or Dallas." I would say, "Mother, there's no family left, just me and you. There's also Shirley, but she is in Pennsylvania and your grandchildren, but all your brothers, sisters and mom and dad are in Kitts Cemetery in Harlan." With that she would settle for minutes and then we would go through the same routine until I took her back to her apartment. At that point she still worked cross word puzzles and I kept her well supplied. I always turned down her bed, placed a crossword puzzle book and a Mr. Goodbar on her bed, helped her into her nightgown and walked her through her apartment checking the doors before leaving. When I got to my car I would also call her and assure her everything was okay and safe. I could always tell by the sound of her voice if she felt secure. If she did not, I would return and go through the procedures again until she was comfortable. Yes, she would spend a few nights with me, but she assured me she always slept better in her own bed. I too slept better when she was in her own bed. Her days were now lost and each waking hour was an existence of another time. Monday no longer had meaning, Sunday no longer meant going to church and she only understood night when it began getting dark saying, "It sure gets dark early now, don't it?" Her world had changed, she no longer felt secure, it would be a change forever, but I pushed myself to make sure she was comfortable and tried to make her happy. A real smile was worth a million dollars to me. It concerned me to think about her fear, but the realization sent chills through me that my mother was partially gone forever in a twisted sort of way, a twisted mind lost in time. Most will live with lots of anger, a feeling of despair, but I challenged my role as caregiver to mother and vowed to make her feel happy without these stressful feelings.

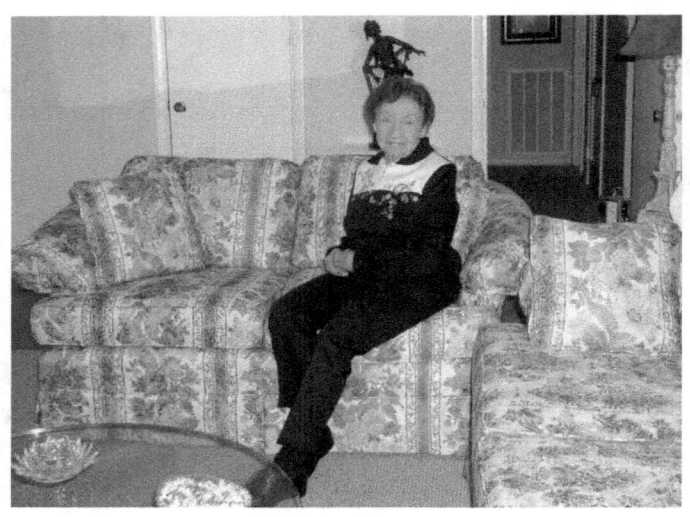

Mother did not look her age. She still had that same youthful appearance, posing for a picture, making sure she looked "just right." Sometimes it was hard for me to think she was in her 80's.

CHAPTER 4 – Dipp'n Gravy

Harlan County, situated in the Eastern part of Kentucky, high in the Appalachian Mountains was known for being very poverty stricken, full of hard living and large families. Food was scarce and stretching a meal included creating variations of gravy, which was a favorite and it stretched the food source enabling a way to feed more mouths. Ms. Emily mastered the art of making apple gravy, tomato gravy, chicken gravy, pork chop gravy, bacon gravy, sausage gravy, bean gravy, blueberry gravy, blackberry gravy and most every kind of gravy you could imagine. Each variation of gravy had a wonderful aroma that made your mouth water while cooking. The smells filled the house. My mother created gravies that were delicious and filling and could have written a book on "How to Make a Meal with Gravy." She could even make fried cabbage gravy with hot succulent buttermilk biscuits. Dipp'n was a way of eating with our meals. We dipped our biscuits, toast, and cornbread. We dipped our fried chicken and pork chops. You could have called us the dipp'n people.

It was Phyllis that first recognized mother's love for this dipp'n. Mother never knew Phyllis was paid to be with her, referred to her as her best friend. Mother was happy again. They had bonded and no doubt Phyllis was a God send for mother, but especially for me. Phyllis introduced mother to the Mexican Restaurant for lunch, ordered their famous Cheese Dip and Nachos. When she introduced Ms. Emily to this new dipp'n, mother looked at Phyllis and said, "This is the best gravy I ever ate." Phyllis laughed hard and passed on the new information, which buckled me with laughter. It became a weekly treat taking mother to the Mexican Restaurant to enjoy their dipp'n gravy.

Sometimes I took Mother for dinner and one evening when the waiter brought the Nachos and Cheese Dip, Mother looked at the waiter and said, "You make the best gravy I ever ate." He could not speak English and looked at me, then back at mother and she said again smiling with a twinkle in her eyes, "You sure make the best gravy I ever ate." He again looked at me with a puzzled look and I could not help but get tickled and she again repeated because he never answered, "You sure make good gravy here." With that, I said, "She likes your food." I sat back enjoying my own private joke. The next day I shared the dinner story to my employees and all who were there. It brought many good laughs knowing how much mother loved Mexican Cheese Gravy.

Often I had good laughs with the food group's mother put together. It was important to her digestive system to have her appropriate food groups daily, but I never knew how she would end up eating these groups. I had seen her dip biscuits into ketchup, French fries into syrup or pour a pack of Sweet N' Low over fried chicken. At Thanksgiving she put Cranberry Sauce on her macaroni and cheese. Not understanding this strange behavior I told a client, an RN, who explained that our sweet taste is the last to go. The elderly will eat anything sweet. I knew mother had a sweet tooth, but pouring all this stuff over good food sometimes unsettled my own stomach.

Mother loved Mr. Goodbars. Phyllis began buying her a bar after lunch; I would buy her a bar as a little daily gift for her bedtime snack not realizing she was stashing Mr. Goodbars all over her house hiding them from me and Phyllis. When I moved mother out of her apartment to live with me, I found Mr. Goodbars wrapped in undies in her underwear drawer, wrapped in a kitchen towel in the towel drawer, hid under sewing material in the sewing box, stashed in the desk drawer, in her night stand, under the mattress and under her pillow. I collected a bag of Mr. Goodbars, along with the socks. We hunted Mr. Goodbars like hunting Easter Eggs. She always stressed that "someone" stole her candy or the "children" ate all her candy, so she made sure she put it in a "safe" place for later. "Why Joyce Ann, if I don't hide my candy someone will get it," she would explain. It was the same for cookies, nuts or candy for the candy dish. I found Oreo cookies in the laundry basket, chocolate chip cookies in her night stand and nuts wrapped in bags with the pots and pans.

During this move I was no longer surprised finding strange things in strange places. In our new home I tried to explain, "Mother, this is the safest home you have ever had and you do not have to hide anything. You don't have to put chairs up against the door or put your shoes up. We have no rats, no children and it is very safe." I could see the thoughts racing through her twisted mind and going out the back door. I knew it was a lost cause trying to make anything stick for more than a moment. Her days were now lost, the span of attention was gone and the task of reasoning with her no longer had meaning. The task of finding ways to communicate and keeping her from becoming irritable came through the "10 Absolutes of Care giving for Alzheimer's Patients." It was also a way for me to have control and it was also a way to save my nerves.

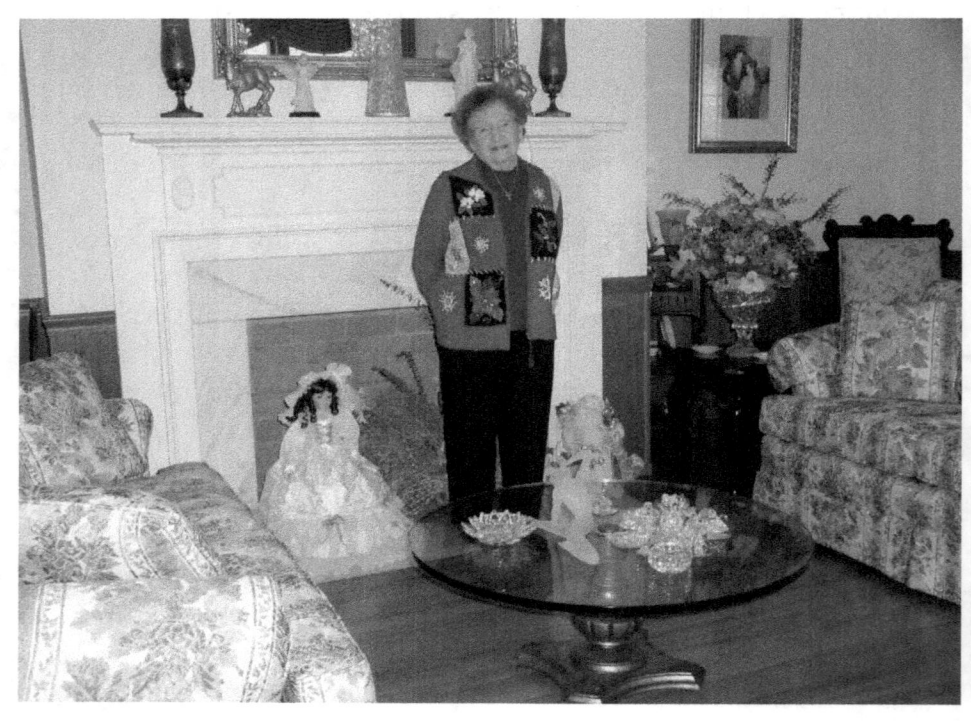

Mother was always happy

CHAPTER 5 – The Naked Lady

My "Little Granny," Dana, my salon manager, began, "loved to go naked. She just hates clothes. Even in the winter time she hates to wear clothes." Dana told the story about one summer day when she and her mother went to Little Granny's house to check on her. "We never called ahead," she said. She proceeded with the story. "Mother and I had a talk about what to expect when we got there, not ever knowing, but this particular day we would be in for a big surprise. We live a couple of miles from Little Granny making the trip very short. The day was beautiful, very sunny and warm and just a slight breeze in the air. When we turned up the little dirt road to Little Granny's house, we continued talking about the usual. What groceries she might need, if we needed to take her shopping for some new clothes and just the usual small talk. As we reached the top of the hill and turned into Little Granny's driveway, there she was hanging out her laundry in "all her glory." I thought my mother would pass out. Of course, I felt a little faint myself, but quickly turned the car off, got out and yelled, "Hey Little Granny, where's your clothes?"

"With that she turned around as if nothing were out of the ordinary and said, "Honey, I am hanging them out to dry!" This was the beginning of our naked lady on the hill. She loved her socks, but she hated those clothes.

It was a funny, funny story, but also had a meaning. What if the weather was cold or rainy? I had heard stories of finding a loved one on the floor naked in the dead of winter. They become lost in their own surroundings and often could find their bed, try to change clothes and become disoriented. Scary, yes and it can break your heart with the thoughts of knowing they were scared and insecure.

These episodes of those suffering from the disease will go from one extreme to the other. Some hate clothes, while others wear layers even during the hottest part of the summer. Temperatures no longer play an important role in the twisted mind, nor does food or the usual daily necessities. There were times I found mother's apartment very hot or very cold. When I tried to explain not to touch the thermostat, it had no meaning. If she became uncomfortable she tried to change the temperature. I resorted to applying tape over the thermostat. It becomes the role of the caregivers' responsibility to make sure their loved one is dressed properly, eats properly and has a safe environment. Bathing could become hazardous, as well as, which includes simple routines such as cooking, or driving. Reverse roles from parent to child, now become child to parent. Remember the old saying, "They revert back to a child." It is true with dementia or Alzheimer's behavior that they no longer are playing the role of parent, but now reverting back to the child. Eating habits change and often the caregiver plays games to get the loved one to finish their meal same as with a child. I found TV was a good tool to use at meal time for mother. She would always say, "I'm just not very hungry, but I am thirsty." I always continued serving the meal, selecting a favorite program for her to watch to distract her while she ate. I urged her to "Try your broccoli," or "This is the best corn bread I ever made." She would take her gaze away from the TV for the moment, pick up her bread or take a bite of another food group without thinking. She was like watching a robot, look at the TV, pick up her food, put it down, watch TV, chew, drink her milk and finally finish her meal.

I continued to encourage another bite until I knew she had had enough. I could tell when she finished as I watched her pile all the leftover food into the center of her plate and cover it with a napkin. She would wrap a sandwich and put it up for later. Cookies could be found wrapped in the cabinet or her nightstand. Food was always protected. I could watch mother and understand her childhood knowing her family had often gone to bed hungry. Never throw food away, she would caution. "Save it for later", she insisted. Yes, she was my child now. I created things to entertain

her, gave her treats, took her to the zoo and made sure she was

safe.

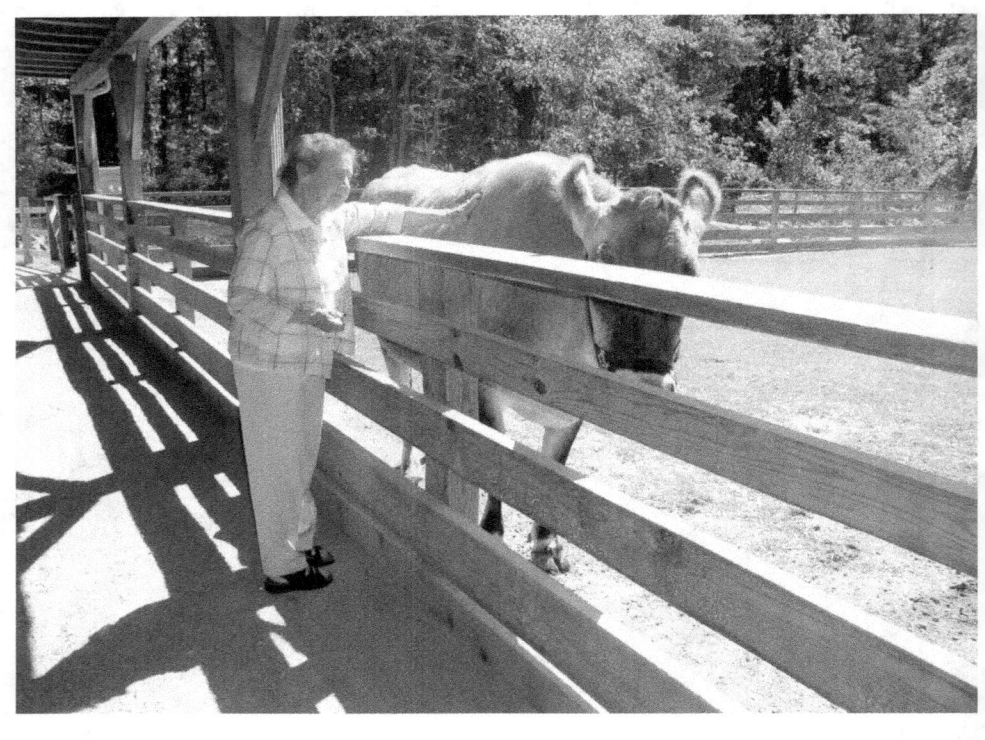

Mother enjoying a fun day at the Birmingham Zoo

CHAPTER 6 – The Golfer

Mother loved her new house. She also loved my clothes. She now had a new house and new clothes, my clothes! She no longer was capable of living alone and I knew the time had come to either put her in a nursing home or move her in with me. I thought my life had changed at the time I brought her to Alabama, and having to care for her, but this was another new experience with caring for mother knowing she was one of the many suffering from dementia. Each day was a new day with a new experience. The simple became the most difficult.

It began with being an ordeal getting mother dressed in warm clothes for the day, but returning from work and finding her in "new" things, my things brought anxiety to me. At this time I had hired no one to stay with mother during the day. It was during this time I also became tired, stressed and wondering if I could continue my role as I had promised never to put mother in a nursing home. Phyllis came on occasion, but not daily.

The first week mother discovered my new beautiful expensive jackets. Each day she found something new and interesting to her lik'n, but to my disappointment. December, this particular year, was especially colder, much more than the weather we had had in previous years. A high of 41 degrees for the day was very unusual, but mother hated seeing leaves on the walk ways to the new house and out she went sweeping after I left for work. I planned her days, knowing that Phyllis would be by to pick her up for her an outing. Phyllis would also call to let me know when she dropped mother Emily back home. I began cutting my day short to be back with mother realizing she should not be alone for long periods of time. Still to my amazement, she could cover a lot of territory in the short two hours she was left alone. By the time I returned home she was into something new out of my closet. My clothes were organized into dress and work clothes in my bedroom closet, golf clothes in the hall closet, coats and jackets in the extra closet and our better dress clothes in the guest bedroom closet.

For some reason mother started getting into my bedroom closet. First it was the fancy sequined jacket and a dinner ring she wore sweeping the front walks, the jacket still had the tags hanging out underneath the arm pits. The next day it was the studded crystal blouse, the next day she had on my new brown pants, rolled up to accommodate her short legs and my brown stripped sweater. Thankfully, she had not discovered the matching belts. The next day she had on my new spring jacket I had purchased on sale at Belk's, and again with the tags still hanging under the arms blowing in the wind as she swept the front walks, all decked out in one of my large diamond and pearl dinner rings. Finally, she had discovered my golf closet and had taken off her beautiful green sweater and replaced it with one of my spring golf sweaters buttoned to her neck. The sweater was somewhat long on me, but when I saw mother in this sweater I could not help but laugh. It came down almost to her little knees. She was so proud of herself and said, "I thought you would like this." At that moment I had to remember how to approach the problem. Remembering the does and don't of handling this disease I remembered, never CONDESCEND, instead, ENCOURAGE OR PRAISE.

Again, I said, "Mother, you look really pretty, but let's change your clothes and get you back into your sweater so we can go shopping. This is my golf sweater and it's for spring and much too cold to wear today. It is almost 35 degrees outside and this is much too light for you to wear. I am proud of you that you like to look very nice." So, off we go to find where she thought she had hung the green sweater. For some reason, the sweater was hung in my bedroom closet, but she had gotten the golf sweater out of the hall closet. To date, I still had not found the girdles or the black velour top.

I knew the routine would not change, but I was happy she enjoyed looking pretty.

Many in this condition will not change their clothing, put on makeup or take a bath. Mother loved sweeping and I had to replace her brooms every three months from sweeping every day. During her stay in the apartment she had accumulated seven brooms. I was sure she took the brooms from the laundry room, or any broom left outside doorways and perhaps she picked up a couple from the back neighbors porches? I will never know. Like the bird bath that mysteriously appeared on her back patio, a beautiful little black iron bird bath, on a pedestal with iron birds perched on the top edge. I could visualize her dragging the thing back to her patio. The day I found it she was sweeping the patio and rearranging her patio furniture I had purchased to accommodate her new treasure. "Where did you get the bird bath," I asked? "I have had this thing for a long time," she answered. Perhaps it came from the back yard of one of the homes in the alley. She loved walking up and down the alley. Said it was her exercise of the day. I would never know how to return the bird bath and felt guilty watching her enjoy it. She had never stolen in her life; it was a form of stealing without knowing. There was no way to change her, but I knew she would have to be watched more closely

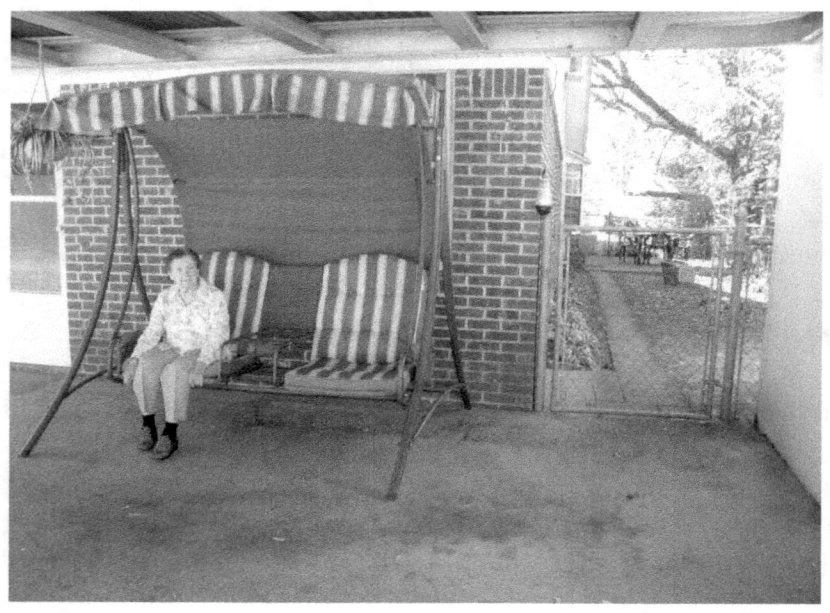

Mother in her apartment with the "bird bath" on the patio

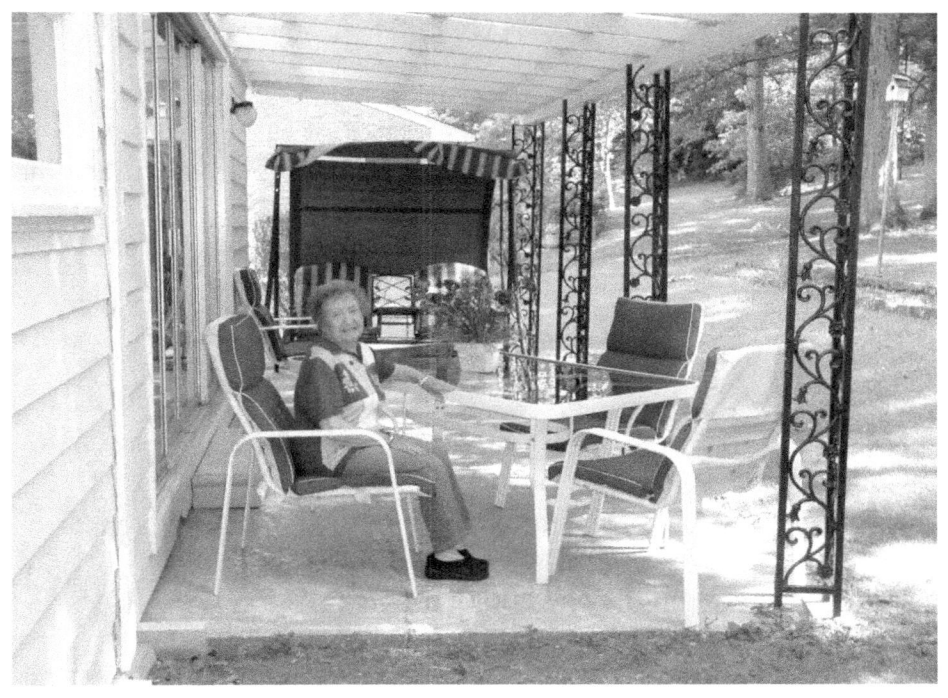

Mother on the patio of her new home and enjoyed visits with the neighbor next door.

CHAPTER 7 – Faster Than Greased Lighting

It was Phyllis's wonderful gentle care with mother that made it possible for me to continue my business trips.   Mother loved Phyllis, but never knew I was paying her to be her best friend. Thank God, Phyllis loved mother as much as mother loved her. This made it easy for me to leave knowing she was in good hands.

During of my trips away Phyllis often expressed her clothes problems she had encountered with mother. One morning Phyllis laid her clothes on the bed prior to her morning shower. When she finished bathing, dried and went to dress she realized her clothes were missing. "Ms. Emily, have you seen my clothes," she called?" "Why no, Phyllis. I can't wear your clothes because they are too big for me." With that Phyllis said mother rounded the corner wearing her bra, top and pants. Gently, Phyllis explained that she probably picked up her clothes instead of hers and retrieved her clothing without confronting mother that she indeed did help herself to the clothing. Phyllis proceeded to help mother find proper clothes out of her own closet, but had learned a good lesson forgetting for the moment that mother no longer had that moment of forgetfulness. Phyllis said she could not help laughing, which annoyed mother, but I too screamed with laughter just visualizing how mother looked in the too long pants, large bra and panties hanging loosely on her tiny body. Phyllis wore a large top because she had long arms, mother wore a small petite. It was almost too funny to imagine how mother must have looked in those clothes, especially the bra.

It was the first of such happenings with clothing, but soon there would be more. Mother had some health issues that had to be addressed and required laser surgery. She was to recuperate in rehab for twenty-one days. It was at that time I moved her, without her knowledge, out of her apartment, to the safety of a larger home I found to accommodate both our belongings. That is when I realized mother could no longer live alone. I decided she would be with me for the remainder of her life or until such time I could no longer care for her.

The nurses at the Rehab Home had fallen in love with her. She visited every room daily, asking if anyone needed anything, but also she helped herself to some of their belongings. I tried to prevent these incidents by allowing her one change of clothing daily. I also changed her into her night clothes, taking her daily wear and leaving a fresh change for the next day. One evening when I began helping her change she did not want to take off her bra. I said, "Mother, this is not your bra!" She protectively held up her hands against her breast and said, "Now Joyce Ann, I like sleeping in my bra and besides this is my most comfortable bra I own." I continued, "Mother, bras bind us and sometimes cause us not to breath properly, sit up and let me unfasten this bra." With that she sat up, I took off the bra and walked over to Florence, her roommate, in the opposite bed and said, "Florence, is this your bra?" Florence burst out laughing and said, "Yes, but that is okay."

I put the bra in her drawer and continued dressing mother in her pajamas.

When I brought mother home from rehab I found a strange pair of men's eye glasses in her makeup bag. Never saying a thing about the glasses to mother, I drove back to the rehab home saying we had forgotten her mirror and slipped the glasses into my coat pocket. When I returned them the nurse said, "These are men's glasses. Now wonder who they belong to?" Everyone in hearing distance laughed as I retrieved mother's mirror and went back to the car.

One morning I missed my favorite black lace bra. After tearing through one drawer, then another, I found it in one of her purses in a drawer along with a Mr. Goodbar. My bra had been laundered the evening before and left on the washer lid to dry, same as the girdle which was never found. I realized I should have learned a lesson by now. Guess I would have to find new places to dry things when mom was up and about. I finally found the black velour top under her blue suede jacket hanging in her jacket closet. Things came up missing and mysteriously reappeared.

I sometimes felt a ghost was following me playing funny jokes and games. Everyday was a mysterious new day. Every mysterious new day brought new rewards, new stress or lots of laughter. Mother always looked so innocent.

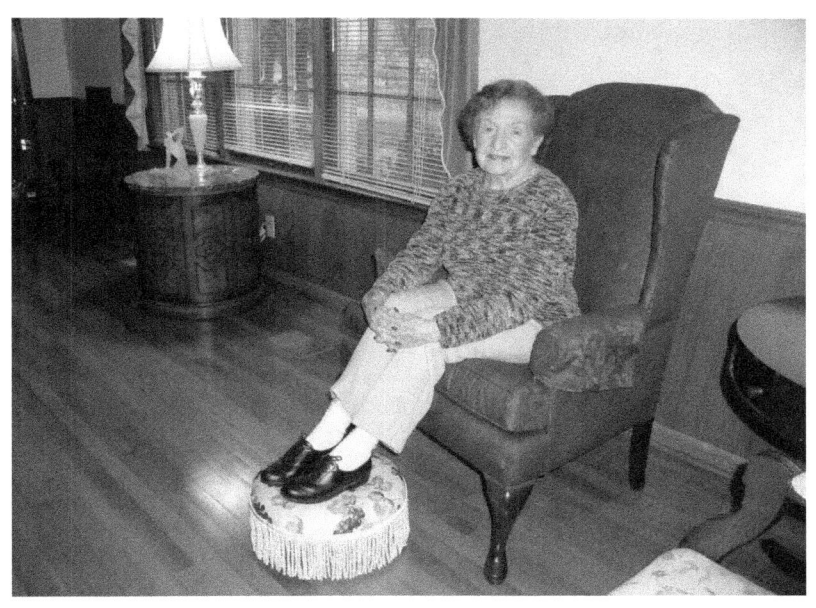

Mother– the face of an innocent child

CHAPTER 8 – Don't Step on the Yellow Line

How do you perceive what happens in the minds of those suffering with dementia or Alzheimer's? Do you question what they do? Do you confront them when they act strangely? Or do you jump on board and ride the train wondering where your ride will take you? As I waited for a new prescription to be filled for mother, and questioned the pharmacist with concerns I had with the side effects, a nurse had sat listening and then she said, "I work with patients and understand what you are going through. It is wonderful to hear someone who works to enforce instead of break down barriers when helping with this disease. It is also important to question medicines prescribed for memory loss. They are not always good for the patient and can carry great risk." Mother had tried the usual memory loss medicine, Arrocept, Excellone and I had heard about another new medicine called Zyprexa. Could it cause nausea, I wondered, or serious side effects? The listed effects definitely made me have concerns, but the pharmacist assured me it was a good medicine with great results. So, I decided to give it a try.

As I waited, the nurse said, "I worked in a nursing home and my favorite patient had dementia. He was the sweetest man I had ever known. At night we lined all the wheelchairs up against the wall along the yellow line. One morning I came to work and all the wheelchairs were on the opposite wall. I stood looking at the chairs. The patient came out of his room and I said, "Why are the wheelchairs on this wall?" He answered my question with assurance as he pointed his finger at the yellow line, "You cannot park on a yellow line," he sternly said. I knew he had taken the liberty to move all the wheelchairs to the opposite wall and said, "Oh, you are right and thanks for catching this before anyone gets into trouble." With that, he smiled, walked back into his room and I could tell he felt constructive with moving the wheelchairs to the opposite wall and off the yellow line before anyone got a ticket. I also realized I had shown a positive attitude with his work. In these homes there is little to do except sit, watch TV and find work. I am sure he felt he had completed his work for the day and was ready to settle down to a nice long nap or watch his favorite TV program."

It was another incident that happened in the same home some time later. A dear friend's husband had placed his father in the home. One of the drawbacks of living in a small town is keeping you in tune with everyone and everyone's business. I had worked with a client with problems stemming from kleptomania. She had had her hands slapped by the law enforcement many times for picking up small items; however, she was the widow of a leading attorney and was left very wealthy. She had also helped herself to small items in my boutique, but I closed my eyes and looked the other way. She had all the comforts of home including maid service. After her husband passed, she developed memory loss and was diagnosed with Alzheimer's. The nursing home had a special ward for these patients, but they were allowed to roam the halls and visit other patients during the day. It was on one of these occasions that my friend encountered the client. It seems a nurse had relayed she was working the desk one morning and engaged in a phone conversation with one of the house physicians. The patient walked up behind the counter, stood behind the nurse, reached over, and with one finger, she pushed down the button on the phone cutting off the conversation abruptly between the nurse and physician. She then stepped back shaking her finger at the nurse, and saying in a very stern voice, "I have told you over and over that you are on my time and my dime and you cannot continue to work for me and talk on my phone. Now don't let me ever catch you on my phone again." With that, she walked off leaving the nurse speechless and stunned.

Remember, arguing is not the answer, but buying into the situation can avoid conflicts that cause high blood pressure, possible stroke or minor problems with nausea associated with stress. We, the caregiver, have to make many changes but the patient no longer has that liberty or privilege. We must look at the situation and instill love, faith and security. These are the things that are valued the most.

When I tucked mother to bed at night the things I said to her with love and affection was, "Mother, you look so comfortable in your soft, cozy bed. I will set your shoes here beside you because in this wonderful house we do not have rats. The doors are all locked and you don't even have to close your bedroom door. I am in the next room. I will turn your nightlight on so you can see if you need to get up. It's so exciting to know we have all those wonderful sensor lights outside. Do you want a glass of milk?" With that, she assured me she was okay then I would kiss her, tuck her in and walk away. I also came back again and said, "Are you warm enough?" When she was secure that I was there, I could see she had settled for the night and I gently walked out giving her one more reassuring smile that I was there forever. She now slept her entire nights without wandering through the house. She no longer tried to put chairs against her bedroom doors. She no longer felt scared, and she knew she was safe with me. She had her food groups, her bath, her medicine and she was in a soft, comfortable bed for sleeping. No, she did not take Xanax or Ambian or any medicines to make her sleep. She knew I would always be there for her. I could tell by the look in her eyes that she was secure. She was now my child. My goal was to care for her and to make sure she felt secure and safe. I did not want her feeling scared as paranoia is a major part of this disease. I did not understand the meaning of how it worked, but I did understand the patience it took to get through the barrier for reassurance. I am not saying it was an easy job, but it was rewarding to know when they felt secure. With that, I too could sleep through the night.

Their strange behavior is much like those of autism. It takes patience to see results. Being repetitious is one of the rules to remember. Keeping the minds occupied and stimulated is very important. Mother had always enjoyed crossword puzzle books. I encouraged her to work these books; however, she went through times she would not pick the books up. I felt she was regressing and asked the doctor if there were new medicines for memory loss. We discussed several medications, some had been tried, which had made her nauseous, but he prescribed Zuprexa. The listed side effects were scary, but as the pharmacist said, "They all have pretty much the same side effects." I decided to give this new one a try. After four days, I wondered if it was just another medicine and perhaps not agreeing with her. I noticed she slept longer hours, but did not notice any other changes. It was Christmas Day when the first signs of something new became visible. She had been on the new medicine for about two weeks, long enough for it to build up in her body. We went to church, stopped off at family for Christmas dinner, visited friends in the rehab center where she had stayed after her surgery and then home to watch a movie. The weather reported snow flurries and we talked small talk of the weather and the events of the day. I kept her crossword puzzle books laid out in her bedroom. I had also bought her a new pair of reading glasses the day before and laid them out on the table beside her chair in my office. She picked up one of the crossword puzzle books, brought it to my office and sat down. I said, "You know mother, really smart people work those puzzles and I am so proud that you are so smart." She smiled, and picked up the book. I said, "Mother, I have pencils sitting there beside the lamp if you want to work your puzzle book." She never said a word, started leafing through her book and picked up a pencil. She continued looking through the book; suddenly I noticed she had begun working her books again. It shocked me that she continued steadily for more than two hours and got them correctly. I wondered if it could be the medicine.

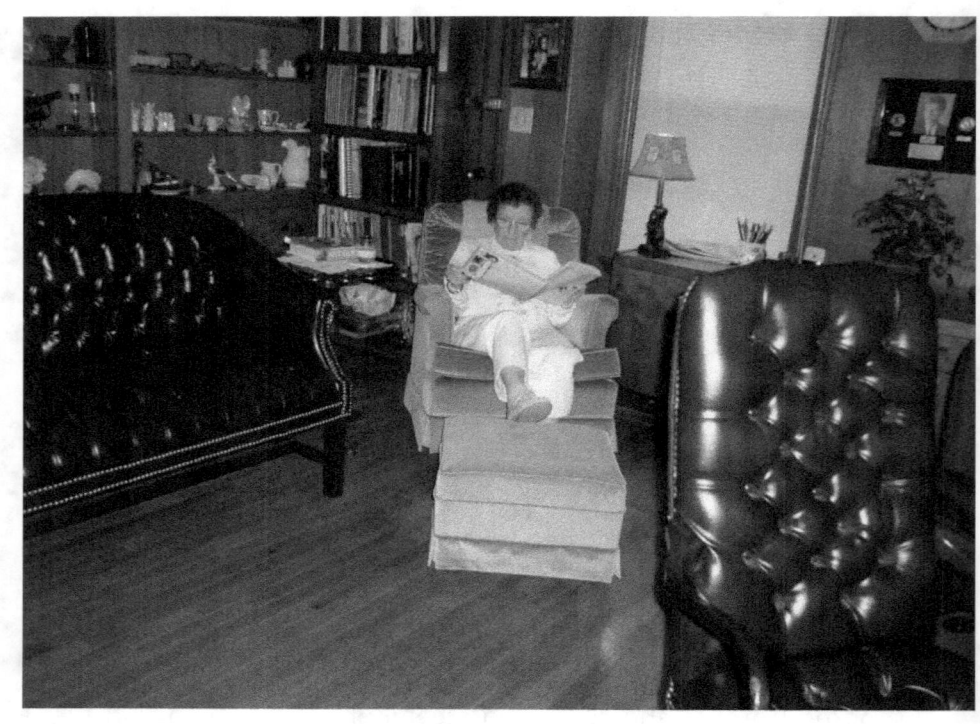

The day Mother worked her crossword puzzle books for more than two hours.

She acted more normal that day than I had seen her in many months. She laughed and teased me even asking if I needed anything and she had teased Florence, her previous roommate, earlier at the rehab center. Florence had relayed a funny story about mother while she was recuperating. "One night," Florence began, "the buzzer from the ankle bracelets some of the patients had to wear kept going off. Someone must be trying to get out the back door." "Well," mother replied, "they just ought to leave them alone and let them escape. It would be one less nut to put up with in this crazy place." We all screamed in laughter. I said, "Florence, I never know what will come out of my mother's mouth". Florence replied, "I had them move me into this private room after Ms Emily left because I was afraid who they may room me up with. I really miss her." Mother said, "Well, you are better off by yourself, but I just may come back, you know."

Unfortunately, the new medicine turned into a nightmare. After several days, she began having reactions and was hospitalized. It started with wandering strangely through the house. She could not settle down and began talking wildly. I even put her to bed with me, but she kept getting up and walking through the house like she was lost. The following day I took her to her doctor. He admitted her to the hospital saying she may have "slid" off the shelf. I did not buy this and felt it was the new medicine. It took weeks for the medicine to wear off. What ensued was a living nightmare and made me realize that my mother was much better off without any medicines. The side effects from the medicine caused her to be disoriented, taking her appetite, made her nauseous, made her do crazy things like rip out her IV's, using the bathroom in the floor, kicking and crying. I knew this was not the usual behavior for my mother and realized the problem stemmed from the medication. The horror from the ordeal made me also realize it could have landed her in the Alzheimer's ward at the nursing home! Older people with dementia cannot express or explain their feelings as the words just do not come anymore. They cannot tolerate many kinds of medication if they are suffering from memory loss, because it can have the opposite reaction. For mother, it was treacherous!

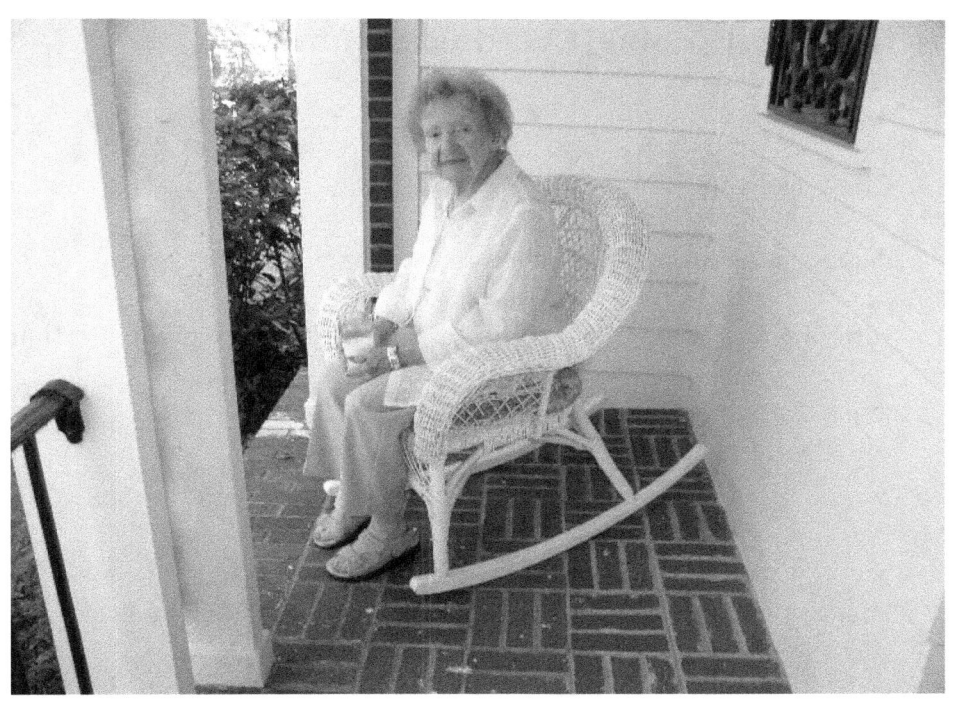

Mother sat on the front porch every morning watching traffic and waving at the people that went by and many that knew her blew their horns and waved. She loved her rocking chair and loved being outside.

CHAPTER 9 - Humor Turns Sad

Often we only look at the humorous side of this disease, but a darker side lurks, untouched by those living inside the body suffering this fate. It is some of the sad sides of dementia that make caring hard for the caregivers.

I began noticing how Mother was making new changes as if she was wilting. Much like a flower, I felt, as I watched her body changes, her gait slowing and hardly cracking jokes. She no longer swept the walk ways or wanted to take long walks in the park. She began talking about being very tired daily. Her eating habits were much the same, but the look in her eyes was changing. I sometimes saw far away looks and the brightness of her eyes were dimming. It was scary to see these changes, but I also realized she was not getting any younger, but fighting Father Time.

The Zuprex backfired on her and landed her in the hospital again. I learned later this medicine had a multimillion dollar lawsuit against it for causing unnecessary deaths. I knew something was happening and began to google her symptoms. Thank God I recognized the symptoms that were caused from the medicine that almost killed her. It took the twinkle away from her eyes and I felt the effects may not be reversible. The medical doctor admitted it was the medicine causing her to act like she had lost her mind. It took weeks for it to get out of her system, but they continued to be visible. The surgery to tack up her bladder did not hold and her fallen bladder was worse than ever. I felt guilty knowing I made the choice to elect cosmetic surgery hoping to give her a better quality of life and I often lay in bed at night crying just knowing this would never change.

During her recuperation in rehab the nurses failed to give her stool softener. Having that old gut feeling, I had called three times in one evening to remind the nurses, but they still failed to give her the stool softener. It was hard to believe a nurse just forgot to give a medicine and it had caused such damage that her lifelong damage could never be repaired. Florence, her roommate, told me what had happened during the night when I arrived the next morning. "Your mother stayed in the bathroom almost all night long and I finally called the nurse," she explained. I realized mother had constipation problems, asked the nurses about the stool softener, but learned they had "forgotten" to give it to her. Angry, yes, but when you are the mercy of rehab centers, there is little one can do. I learned later it was permanent damage as her bladder had broken back down from all her straining during the long night. She had gone through all the surgery for nothing! If you fight with these people they will not take the care needed for the patient. Both the bladder and the uterus had torn back down which left her in worse shape than ever. Yes, it was permanent. "God," I thought, "How could this rehab center forget to give a new patient, just out of surgery, stool softener?" I cried until I was nearly sick myself when I realized what had happened, but it was too late. It also made me realize that my mother was just another old woman in their facility. She was at their mercy and there was little I could do.

Months passed trying to deal with the problem. Ulcers formed on the bladder which now hung outside her body the size of a golf ball and rubbed against her clothing. It also made walking for any distance difficult preventing our long walks in the park or full days of shopping. I finally bought little panty girdles that seemed to help some and when we would go shopping we would get a wheel chair. She was so vain at first not wanting to get into a wheel chair, but with Kimberly's help we finally coaxed her into trying it at Walmart and she loved it. After that day she never minded riding in a wheel chair. Even with the dementia, she still had lots of pride and would tell you in a heartbeat that she could walk by herself.

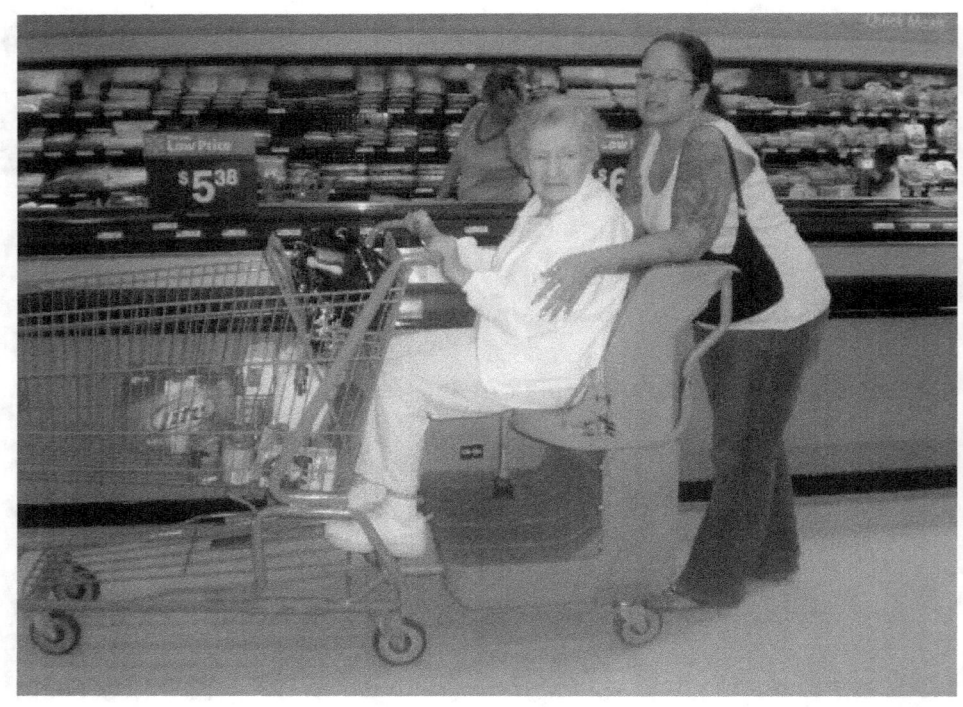

Both our lives had now changed. It would limit anything we did away from the comforts of home. The bladder could not empty properly causing mother to need relief facilities often. We were also limited to long trips we enjoyed on occasion. Mother had a miserable life now because of the careless care given her in the rehab center. I also realized you could not depend on these homes without the family's good care and love and attention. When I questioned this, the answer I received was, "We are short of help."

What could we do?

Some months later, my poor Mother fell and broke two ribs in the kitchen. When she fell she fell straight down to the floor and bruised the bladder now hanging outside her little body. It stayed very swollen, and she developed a serious urinary tract infection plus having to deal with the ulcers on her protruding bladder. She could no longer do her exercise to keep it in place. It was hard to understand how she walked in this shape, but being the trooper she was, she did not complain and walked very slowly. Mother was not a candidate for another major surgery and somehow managed to live with this horrible problem caused by a negligent nurse. I soon learned that a caregiver also had to make sure their loved ones was cared for and not depend on hospital personnel or nursing home staff. You had the right to read their charts and question their medicines. These homes are usually overloaded with patients and staffs that do not have the time to give personal care. I took mother out of this center after 11 days. I gave her better care than what her Medicare paid for, which was a full 21 days of paid care. It could have given me some off time, but I could not rest knowing she was not properly being cared for.

At the beginning of my memoirs I talked about how Mother became lost inside herself because of losing her daughter, so tragically. To add to her many problems, the tides had turned making her lost in her surroundings. She was born and raised in those beautiful mountains of Eastern Kentucky, now she was having to live in another state, in another house and her surroundings were no longer familiar with her. This too, added to the dementia problems. She had wandered from our home on four different occasions, but the last brought me to my knees and I begged God to allow me to find her in good health and unharmed.

It was Mother's Day, 2006. We were scheduled to attend a family reunion in Townley, AL with my father's people, the Romine's. Every morning I tried to catch mother before she had time to dress herself, but this particular morning she had awakened, dressed and was ready for the day. Strange but she had on her "new" outfit I told her she could wear for this special day.

The first indication that the day would not go well became obvious when I mentioned taking a shower and changing clothes. Mother was very self-conscious about her appearance and her hygiene. It would embarrass her to make her feel she had not "washed up." Even when I approached the subject delicately, it never came across to her that I was not suggesting she was dirty. In her mind, she had already bathed. It was most always a fight with the shower thing. I made sure I stayed with her during the shower and making sure she did not fall. Later I began bathing her myself. Even when standing with her, she almost fell one morning. This could be disastrous which could break her hip or bones.

On this particular morning I had her Mother's Day gifts wrapped and waiting with a fresh cup of coffee. Knowing I would have a problem I suggested she change and "let's get our shower before we had coffee." I could tell she was angered, but I thought it worked, but while I was preparing her bath, she quickly changed, slipped out the back door and was gone in a matter of minutes.

First I thought she was in the guest bathroom, but after carefully searching through the house, I knew she was gone. She usually went next door, but the maid said she had not seen her. I asked everyone walking the park and no one had seen her. I thought I heard her voice at one time from the woods, but when I went in the direction of the sound I could not find her. I drove the streets several times before calling 911. With the wonderful help of the rescue squad and the police, mother was found after 1 1/2 hours and almost three blocks away not knowing where she was. By the time she was found, I was sick with fright. I visualized everything and knew she was not strong from the broken ribs she had suffered a few weeks prior plus it was very hot and I thought about her having a heat stroke. She told the police she thought I was mad with her. I held her in my arms, cried and told her of course I was not angry and assured her of my love. We made the family reunion, but my blood pressure was so high and my day was ruined. By evening she had not remembered anything, including our day in Townley. As we sat and watched TV that night, I knew I had to make yet another change for her safety. So Monday I immediately took mother to the police department and had them apply a monitoring bracelet on her ankle.

I did not intend to go through another day like Mother's Day 2006. When the police found her she told them she could not find her house. When they brought her home she said she thought I did not want her. As I held her in my arms crying, I tried to make her realize I always wanted her. The mind is strange, but the behavior is stranger with this horrible disease. Thank God Mother was okay, but the effect it had on her badly fallen bladder would never heal. I will never get over my hurt for knowing how she must have felt for 1 1/2 hours walking the streets that were unfamiliar to her. I thought about her fear and the pain in her ribs. I thought about the heat and how her bladder must have hurt. I thought about her feet now plagued with bunions and thought about how quick she had slipped out of my sight. I thought I was in control of my mother, but I now realized I had to make double sure she would be safe for the rest of her life. As the old saying goes, "they revert back to childhood," and it really is very true. She was now my baby. I often dreamed of taking her shopping and losing her. For many weeks I woke up in a sweat listening for her door to open and often checking to see if she was still in bed. My nights were no longer restful for fear of what the stillness of the night might bring by dawn. She was in my care.

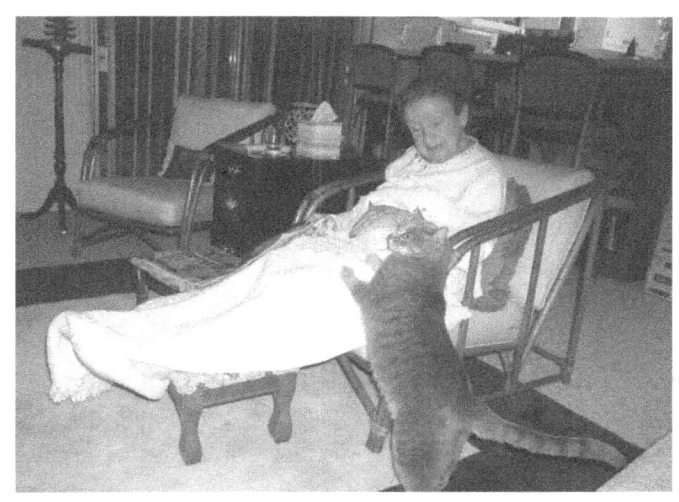

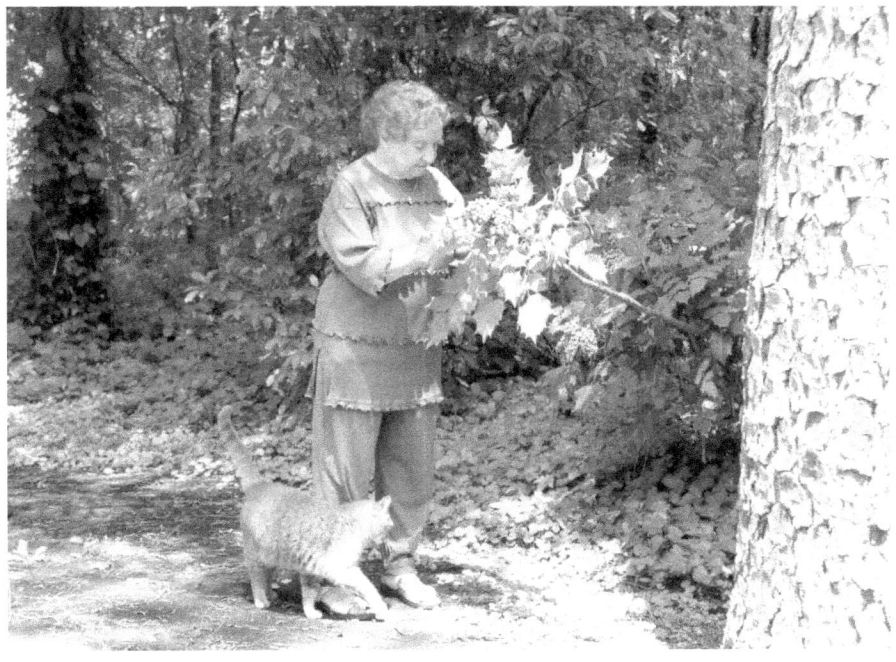

Mother and Tabatha

CHAPTER 10 – Are You Hungry?

Mealtime had always been a very special time in our family. It was a time we were all together and enjoyed conversation. We began by holding hands making a circle while my father offered thanks for our food. It continued, but at this time of mother's life, she became the child, I became the mother but, she continued to pray thanks as we held our circle of hands. It was like an automatic thing when we were ready to eat. When we went to restaurants we always reached across the table and held hands as she said her special prayer.

This particular morning I watched as she sat in her rocking chair gazing out the sunroom watching the squirrels and birds. Her eyes were happy and she was content. She knew I cared for her in every sense of the word. Daily, she told me what a wonderful daughter I was and how lucky she was. I looked at her as she sat content with her surroundings, very quiet as though she were lost in time, perhaps thinking of her life on the mountain in Harlan County, or about daddy or my dad. I never knew what she was thinking anymore. It was a challenge to keep her occupied while she ate and I tried to cook food as she sat there making the aroma of the bacon and eggs fill the air thinking she would turn to me and say, "Oh, boy, Joyce, that smells good." Those words never came anymore, so I always made a big deal out of each meal, "Mother, are you hungry," I began. She would answer always say yes and then I would say, "Gosh, we have a wonderful meal." Once we sat down at the table, if her chain of thought was broken, she would fiddle with her food, and then I knew she was finished and no need to try to get her to eat more.

First the food must smell good and second it must look good. Mother was small and large portions made her feel sick. I loved taking her to restaurants with food bars so she could choose her own foods. Food groups are important to the elderly because of their digestive system which does not react as it did when they were younger. Without proper food groups daily, they become constipated, develop bowel blockage and the ultimate can happen. A simple routine could make their life easy or complicated.

Mother's days were filled mostly with enjoying the walking, never taking a nap, but always moving and staying busy. My meals were planned daily and I had already planned for stir fry steak and vegetables with yellow rice and cookies for desert with a glass of cold milk for dinner that night. A simple meal with all the right food groups made for the ending of a good day. After dinner we would retired to my office, making sure she was cozy in her reclining chair to watch her favorite TV program, "America's Funniest Videos." She loved this program, but always refused to go to bed. I then switched to CNN and I would watch her out of the corner of my eye while working on my computer as she slowly settled down and gently went to sleep in her chair. Once she was totally relaxed, I gently woke her and told her it was time for bed. She never refused going to bed once she had settled down. This made me realize they have to relax before going to bed alone. It reverts back to the security they need, but once relaxed they were easy to maneuver and coax.

Dementia and Alzheimer's patients always get scared when the sun starts to go down. It is called, "Sun downing." Mother showed little signs of this because I tried to make her feel safe, secure and comfortable. As the sun went down each day, I immediately closed the curtains and turned on the TV keeping her preoccupied. Simple task, like closing the drapes, made her feel safe and secure for the evening. Each night I walked her to her bedroom, took her to the bathroom, tucked her into bed, kissed her goodnight and turned her lights off letting her know I was right there with her. Lucky for me, mother slept through most of the nights. Most dementia or Alzheimer's patients wonder through the house at night, lost in another world.

When mother first moved in with me she also wondered through the house during the night, but with lots of love, affection and reassurance that everything was locked and secured, she slowly melted into my arms and trusted that I had everything secure for the night. Could you imagine being scared every night of your life? Not me. And I did not intend to allow my mother to have those scary feelings. Yes, it was hard, but she was the only mother I would have and I knew she would not be with me forever.

Bird feeders in the back yard kept her attention during the day and she loved watching the squirrels climb the feeders eating the bird food. Often, I put Vaseline or WD 40 on the pole. She laughed so hard just watching them when they tried to climb the pole; holding on for dear life, looking around and then slid back down. They would go farther back from the pole, run harder, and try to grab hold higher on the pole, but with the slick surface I had greased up for them, they came sliding back down each time. We both howled with laughter. I often told her that I must video our backyard zoo so she could send it to our favorite TV show. Patience, love and

attention was required for those suffering this dreadful breakdown

of the brain. How many of us could survive without TLC?

CHAPTER 11– Where is my phone, Mother?

Most days were typical beginning with breakfast, shower, makeup, hair and settling down to the backyard zoo. Phyllis came every Tuesday and Thursday, while Debbie stayed Monday, Wednesday and Friday. I had the weekend. Both sitters knew to keep their car keys out of sight from mother, their purse, anything that was not nailed down could be picked up in a second and tucked away in some "safe" place in her bedroom. This was typical of one with dementia. Once, when Phyllis had her cell phone in her pocket, but forgot to put it in a safe place while I was away on a business trip, she carelessly laid it on the counter in the kitchen while cooking. As the day progressed Phyllis later told me she began hunting her cell phone. She realized she had not put it back in her pocket. The quizzing began, "Ms. Emily, have you seen my cell phone?" "Why, no Phyllis, I haven't seen your phone." The hunting continue from room to room, first in the sofa thinking it may have dropped out of her pocket.

The house was combed, but the cell phone did not show up. Phyllis then began beeping for the phone. She could faintly hear the sound, but could not find where it was coming from as mother helpfully trailed long, being so close that Phyllis backed into her. Finally, she went to mother's bedroom with mother right along behind her trying to detect where the sound was coming from. She decided it was coming from mother's chest of drawers, being the typical hiding place for all mother's cherished possessions. As she leaned next to the drawers, straining and keening her ear to hear the beep, mother was right there close to her side tentatively leaning over while Phyllis was trying to listen. As Phyllis leaned down closer to the side of the chest, she realized the beeping was coming from mother's pants pocket. Mother had the cell phone in her pocket the whole time. I was sure she watched Phyllis put the phone in her pocket many times having the same thought that this would be a good place for the phone. Later we had a good hearty laugh thinking about mother following Phyllis from room to room hunting the cell phone all the while having it in her own pocket. We both knew this would not be the last time for hunting missing items.

Strange how mother did not get into my purse, bother my keys, never took anything out of my office, but if it was from someone that did not live in the house she seemed to be drawn to their belongings. It had nothing to do with stealing, but more of infatuation with something "new" in the house. It was the way their minds worked, which made it hard to understand. A jacket over a chair could end up hanging in mother's closet. A purse could end up in her chest of drawers. Sun glasses could be found in her dresser drawer with her eye glass case. Cookies, months old, could be found wrapped up in a drawer along with peanut butter and jelly sandwiches. Keys could be found in her jewelry box. The list could go on and on. Girdles may never be found.

Once I found the iced tea pitcher in the formal dining room sitting in an antique bowl on the server. Another time, I found the toilet tissue I had purchased beside the desk in the great room; pajama's hanging up, my shirts in her nightstand or the broom in the corner of the formal living room.   You dealt with what you had to deal with. You made the best of the days and listened to the same stories over and over, but you never argued or disagreed. Phyllis and Debbie both understood mother as I did. Mother loved them both and I trusted them to care for her while I was away on business. They also helped relieve me of tension that built up from caring. Unless you had been there, you could not understand the stress it caused, but I also could never put mother in a nursing home. It was worth all the stress to have her with me. Sometimes I laughed, sometimes I cried, but when I tucked her to bed at night she looked at me with those beautiful hazel blue eyes and told me how much she loved me and appreciated me and it melted me.

Holidays were special and as she had made them for me growing up, I made them for her. We always did something special on the 4th of July and one year Phyllis invited us to celebrate with her family at her daughter's home on Smith Lake. Mom and Phyllis both had their 4th of July outfits on. I knew not to get her clothes out the night before, but those were the times I closed her door and wondered if I would see those hazel blue eyes the next morning.

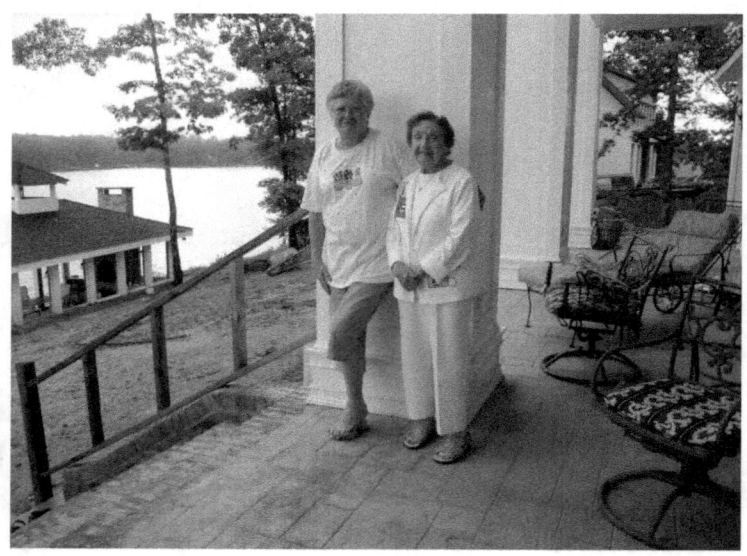

Phyllis and Mother at Yolanda's on the 4th of July

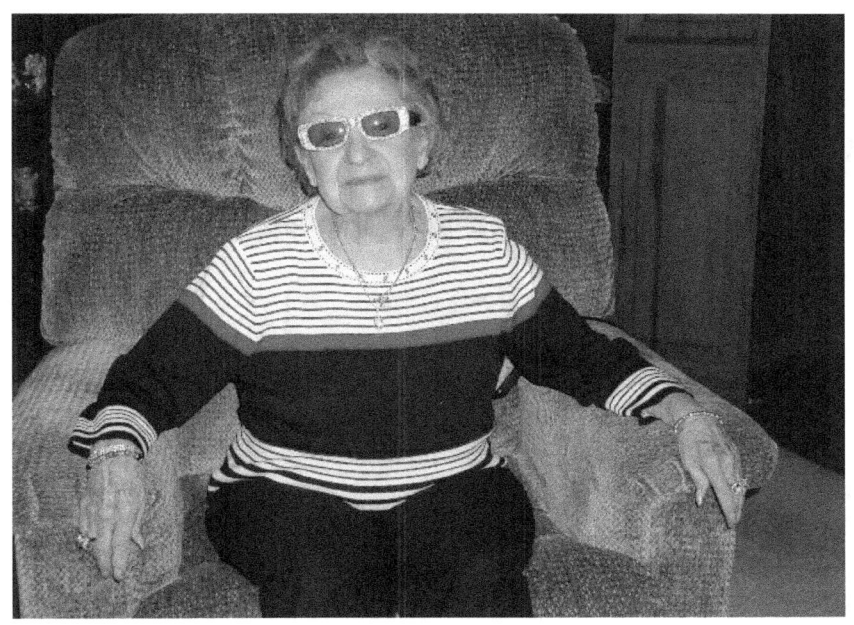

Later that day at home she found her fancy "Hollywood" sunglasses.

CHAPTER 12 – Another Blue Day

Weekends were most always the same. I kept the housework up during the week except for some of the ironing. My first priority was getting mother's breakfast, shower, dressed, makeup and hair done before I decided my next chore of the day. It was a beautiful Saturday morning and I gave mother the leftover cornbread to crumble to the birds. She loved to feed the birds and out the back door she went. I had the ironing board up so I could watch her out the back window. She crumbled the cornbread and casually walks around the yard.

I thought little about what she was doing and continued working. First she went to the upper end of the yard and casually looked at some of the new flowers just popping out of the ground. I enjoyed watching her have fun in the yard. Her life was built around being outside, roaming the mountains as a child and clearing land for a new garden. As I continued to watch her, I knew the wheels were turning that morning, but I had no idea what direction they were going. Obviously, I was not on that train of thought with her.

I continued to iron several pair of pants and shirts, took them to the bedroom to hang up and back to the kitchen. Suddenly, I noticed I could not see mother anywhere. Opening the back door I called, no answer. I then went to the front door and called, but no answer. I then panicked, ran to my bedroom and quickly changed into shorts and top. I ran out the back door and started screaming for mother. After several loud screams the back door of the neighbor's house opened and there mother and the maid stepped out. She had gone "visiting" again. For some reason it shattered my nerves. My blood pressure always shot up sky high when she slipped off and it took days for me to recover. I rarely cried anymore, but for some reason when she walked away and I could not find her it always seemed to bring on a flood of tears. My heart pounded so hard it felt like it was coming out of my chest, my mouth went dry; I shook with fear and prayed for her safety. It was now the fifth time she had left the house.

My thoughts were constantly on how to make my home safer for mother and thought about putting the ankle bracelet back on, but her skin was so thin and fragile the width of the bracelet left scabs on the back of her little ankle. I also realized that she was capable of leaving in a split second and all but running to put away the clothes that morning was not fast enough to know what her mind had decided to do next. It kept me on my toes every minute. Bathroom duties or shower duties were difficult for me. I decided to put motion detectors above the doors to let me know when she went in and out of the house. What do you do with a grown child? At least she could not reach high enough to turn the door alarms on or off.

I take mother by the hand and gently lead her back to the house explaining that she cannot leave without letting me know where she is going. She said, "Why Joyce Ann, that woman motioned for me to come over there." Of course, it was a figment of her imagination. The maid smiled and mentioned mother knocking on the back door so she let her in. At least everyone in this small town knows my mother, but if we lived in a big city I would be a nervous wreck. I wondered how others coped with the same situation.

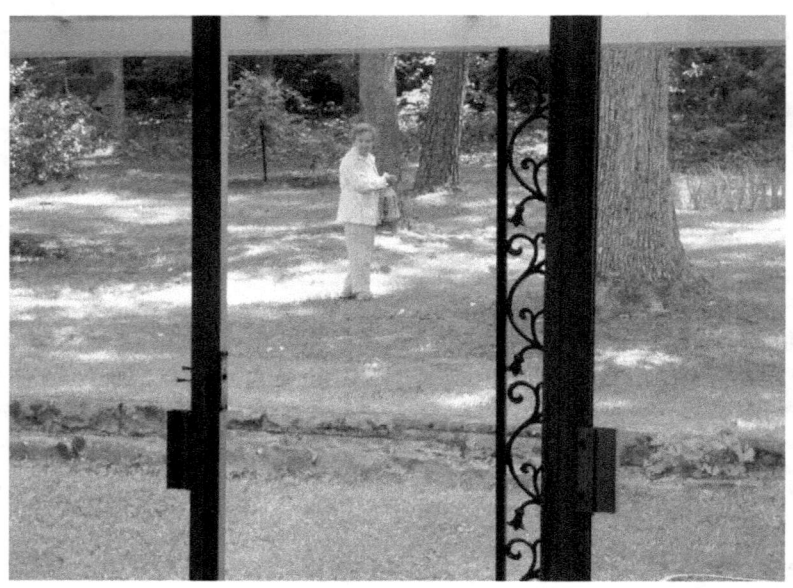

Mother feeding the squirrels and birds and quick as a flash she is

go

CHAPTER 13 – Spoiled Milk

"Mother, your granddaughter is moving next door. Do you remember Kim," I asked. She replied, "Of course I remember Kim, Joyce Ann. What do you think that I've done gone crazy?" With that I left well enough alone. Kim lived in Orlando, Florida, but with a recent life threatening scare made her decide to move to Alabama. We had worked a trade show in Vegas promoting my new product for the esthetic/medical market. When she returned to Orlando she was robbed and beaten near to death. Fortunately the house on the other side of me had been empty for months and I offered this to her in exchange for moving here, putting Christy into college and giving her a salary position in the company. She had already given it thought, had discussed the move with Christy and I immediately went to the real estate company and got the house.

It had been a hard day for Kim to drive from Orlando bringing her first load of small stuff, dishes, clothes, items she could get in her SUV. We unloaded the car the evening she arrived and spent the next day picking out furniture and accessories. I put steaks on the grill, cooked corn on the cob, baked potatoes and had ice-cream and cake for desert. Mother had enjoyed the day, but I could see she was very tired. She loved helping with the kitchen, putting her milk back in the refrigerator and clearing the table. After dinner I did the usual putting mom down for bed. Kim and I stayed up talking and having fun researching the pit bull breeders on the computer. She raised pit bulls professionally and it was from her love for these beautiful dogs that she was robbed.

A young man came by her house asking if she had any pit bulls for sale. Kim replied she had two puppies. He then asked if he could see the puppies and she took him through her home to her kennels and showed him her puppies. He chose one, told her he would have to get his money, he left. Thinking he had gone to his car, she waited until he returned. He then paid, asked if she would get the chosen puppy out of the kennel. She replied, "Of course." With that she bent over the kennel and he put a gun to her head. He stripped her of all her jewelry, much of it heirloom handed down from the family. He pistol beat her first, then drug her by the hair of the head to her bedroom demanded more money and threatened to kill her. She fought for her life, finally breaking lose and running to the neighbor across the street screaming. They first thought she had been shot from all the blood and they called 911. The police and rescue also thought she had been shot, but when they got her to the hospital they realized her head had been split open, he had bitten her extremely bad on her right wrist, on her back and the back of her leg. He also kicked her so intensely he left his footprint in her chest, blackened her eyes, plus multiple bruises and scratches.

Kim's life was changed forever and it left her very scared and depressed. She kept it from me for two days, but I had strong premonitions and finally she told me what had happened. I had offered the house previously, but she declined saying she did not like Jasper. She now realized that Orlando was full of crime and drug problems. Thank God Christy was not in the house at the time. We both felt he would have killed one or perhaps both had she been home. The robber is still at large, but he had robbed five other homes in the same neighborhood prior to hitting Kim's.

We sat enjoying looking at the beautiful pit bull puppies one day when Kim decided to have milk and cookies. She went to the kitchen, opened the cabinet and lifted out a cup for her milk. As she tilted the cup she realized it was full of milk. Soured milk! Mother had put her cup of milk in the cabinet next to the refrigerator and it poured all over Kim. Goodness, it smelled awful. She shrieked trying to ward off the milk, but it had poured all over her nightgown and faintly into her hair. She looked at me and said, "Mother, what is soured milk doing in the kitchen cabinet?" I said, "Kim, this is only the beginning. You know mother. When she gets tired she gets confused and I am sure she put the milk up in the cabinet thinking it was the refrigerator." We both just broke down and laughed. I think she was getting the message what to expect from mother.

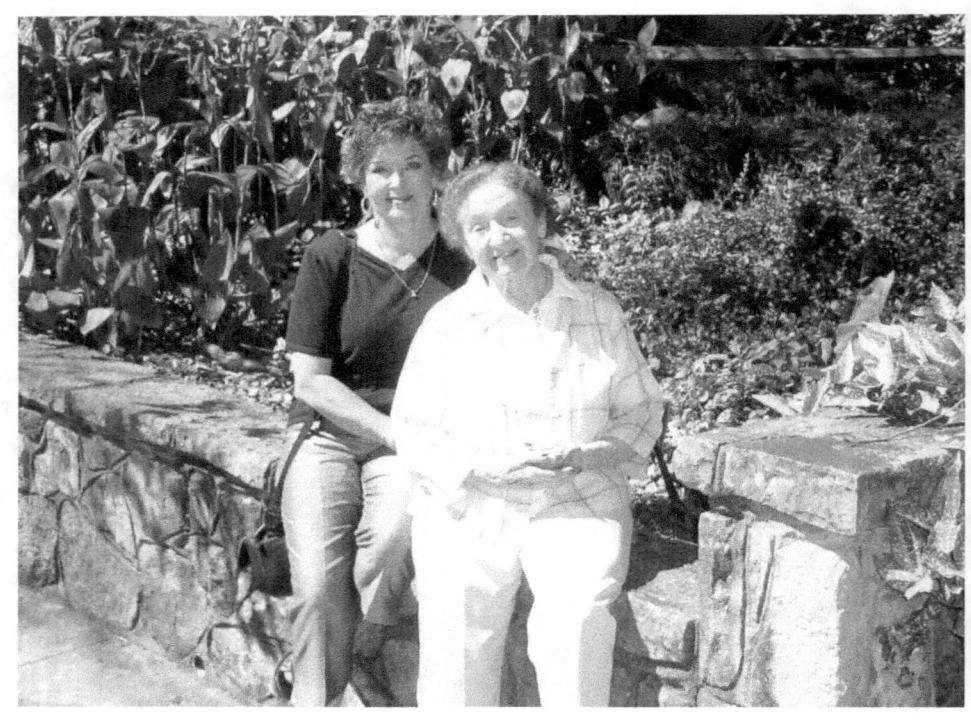

It was a challenge to keep up with her every move.

CHAPTER 14 – Sitters

The days were difficult trying to get mother ready before the sitter's arrival each day, but some sitters could add to the difficulty of the problem.   The first sitter loved mother, but she was now in a nursing home as a stroke left Ollie Mae in a wheelchair and others to care for her. She was missed by both me and mother; however, we took time to visit her. She was younger than mother and it was sad to see her in this shape.

The second sitter was Phyllis, a wonderful friend to mother. She worked part-time, but dependable when I ran into an emergency. She was the kind of sitter that wanted to be part of mother's life, keep up with her health, went with me when mother had to go to the hospital and gave her lots of TLC. I was always comfortable knowing Phyllis would be spending nights with mother when I was away. The third sitter fussed with mother, kept her nervous, called me on business trips complaining that mother would not let her do this or that and I finally had to let her go. Her stay was short lived when she complained about mother. She relayed angrily to me that while out on the back deck "cutting her toenails," mother was busy hiding her purse. I explained, "Betty, you deserve to have your purse hidden if you left mother alone in the house. You are fortunate you could find your purse. I still could not find the two girdles." With that I paid her, asked for the key back and she left. Mother returned to her old self, with the exception, of course, the mind did not return, but I could deal with her. She no longer became agitated and when I came home she no longer took me aside and said, "I don't like that woman. I wish she would leave. She tries to boss me and tell me what to do"

The fourth was Doris. Mother complained from the beginning that she smelled and could not stand her cigarette smoke. Even though Doris smoked outside the house, she still had the smoke smell. When she spent nights with mother, the extra bedroom bed linens smelled of smoke. I also found cigarette butts in the rocking chair in the guest bedroom. She had no car and her husband had to bring her to work daily. She had no phone which made it difficult to contact her for scheduled changes. She was honest and I knew she cared for mother until she took a second job with the Wal-Mart Super Center. One morning when she arrived for work I had asked her husband how many hours she slept prior to coming to care for mother. He replied, "About hour." Then I began feeling she was sleeping on the job because of changes I began noticing. I felt she was gouging me with money when she charged me almost $900 for a few days while I was away on a business trip. I had also used Phyllis during those same days and the expense was much higher than I had planned paying both for the week I was away.

I should never have asked this sitter to do anything for me other than care for mother, but I broke down and asked for help. I rented the house next door for my daughter and granddaughter. I asked if my sitter's husband wanted to clean the yard and clean the gutters. That was another hefty $210. I had hired a professional yard man to do my yard which only cost $75 and he had spent an entire day working. When I questioned this, she became irritated and would not back down saying they both had worked hard and charged me by the hour. I explained that yard work was not an hourly wage. I had never paid a yard man hourly, but for the job. I paid, but felt uneasy. When I came home unexpectedly after taking mother to Birmingham for a doctor's appointment, I found her inside my house helping herself to cold drinks! That also made me feel uneasy knowing she entered my home while I was away without asking.

There were many times I dropped in unexpectedly and found this same sitters husband at the house and on one occasion I called home from a business trip and heard children and adults talking in the background. When I asked who was there, she replied, "Her daughter and granddaughter." She continued that they had dropped by to visit. When I learned her husband had spent an entire week at the house I explained that she needed to tell him this was a job and he should go home and return only when it was time to pick her up. I found them both smoking outside while mother was left alone inside.   During this time I noticed a change in mother. She would have different clothing on when I returned home from work. I would find my clothes folded in her chest drawers along with the towels. I found her good pants I had ironed folded in other drawers in her room and looked for days for the new case of toilet paper I left in the kitchen.

On one particular day I started out trying to get mother's shower, makeup, hair fixed and breakfast that ended in a nightmare. I had purchased mother a beautiful new green blouse, kami and pants to match for special occasions. That morning I left her in Capri's and matching top. Susie knew about the new outfit and that I did not want mother wearing it for every day wear. When I returned mother was in the green outfit which made me upset. She attacked me with, "Your mother has nothing to do all day and if she wants to put on a different outfit it is okay." I replied, "It is not okay when I buy her clothes, leave her in your care and ask that she not wear her new clothes for everyday." She came back with, "She can wear anything she wants because she is an adult." I came back with, "You are right, but I make the decisions for her and that is why you are here. You are on my time and my dime and you are paid to do what I ask of you." She replied, "I don't have to do anything you tell me to do. I even helped her change into that outfit." That statement made me furious, but I still held my ground. With that she got up in my face full of anger and began cursing saying that I showed my a - - every day when I came home. I asked her to get out of my face, but I could see she would not back down. I then said, "Well, if you won't get out of my face, I will get out of yours, but if you work for me you will have to comply with my directions and care for my mother as I have asked. I pay you, mother does not." She said, "If you don't like what I do, you can get someone else." I said, "Good, if that is what you want, but you need to decide if you don't want to work for me anymore.

I stood and looked at this woman and continued, I feel there is very little you have to do in my home other than give my mother 100% care while you are here. I don't leave you with a dirty house or work to do." She said, "No, I don't want to work here anymore and you can cut my check and I will not be back." I explained I would be happy to cut her check the next day, but had left my checkbook at the office. The incident left me drained. Poor mother stood there as this girl attacked me with her vicious words. I kept our house clean, all the laundry done, cooked all the food and all she had to do was to entertain mother, take her for short walks at the beautiful park across the street and make sure she did not rearrange everything in the house. I was happy the day this girl left and again, mother returned to as normal as could be expected. Strange, but I could always tell when a sitter did not do their job. I could always tell when I needed to find a new sitter and I knew this was one of those times. Mother hated cigarettes and had complained that she smelled. It was pleasant to come home and not smell cigarettes in the house or worry about mother's care.

Often on the weekends Kim and I would take mother shopping with us. We talked about how her memory was fading and I knew she seemed to have some trouble seeing things. Often she saw things we knew were all in her head. It was Saturday and we decided to go to the Galleria in Birmingham to shop. Mother loved shopping, but she was getting very slow. We never minded taking more time to shop with mother, but this particular day became one we both would always remember and laugh until we buckled each time it was brought up. Kim and I loved talking and mother loved watching people and walking, but as we walked through the mall I noticed mother was stepping very high. I kept pulling her and saying, "Mother, come on," as I held her hand. I could feel her stopping along, finally asking her what she was doing. "I am stepping over the fences, Joyce Ann," she said. "What fences, mother? There's no fences in this mall." She said, "Just look," and pointed down to the floor. I realized she was stepping over the squares as we crossed each one. Kim got tickled and I tried to keep her from stepping so high, but it was useless. She continued stepping very high over each crack in the squares of the tiled floor. Finally Kim said, "Mother, get her over here where there's no squares." With that I pulled mother to the side of the mall and continued walking, but we were laughing so hard we could hardly walk or talk. Mother jumped right in and laughed with us never knowing what we were laughing about. Mother had cataract surgery in one eye a good while before that day and I later realized she was having floaters in her eyes and was seeing black lines making her think the squares were fences. There was never a dull day with mother. Then I found Sopie, a real love.

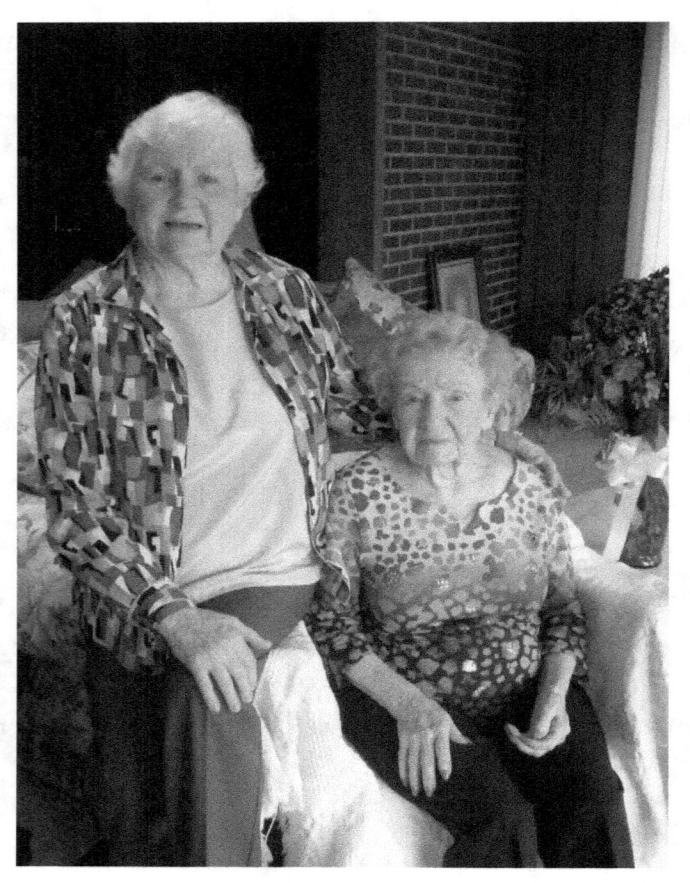

CHAPTER 15 – Graveyard or Golf Course?

The first signs of fall were everywhere. A little breeze, no humidity, a beautiful Sunday and it was Mother's 87th birthday, September 3, 2006. She would quickly tell you she was born September 3, 1919, had all her teeth and still did all her housework, even though she enjoyed sweeping the front walk once in a while, but did make her bed the minute her tiny feet hit the floor. She was quick to go brush her teeth and wash her face, but as time progressed with the memory loss, she would tell you she had done all the above. Now I made the effort to get this done for her, except I would stand and make sure she brushed her teeth well.

I had not played golf since my friend, Betsy, passed June 12, 2004 of Pancreatic Cancer and also Carrie, breaking up my foursome. All my friends had their little foursomes now leaving me alone to play. I continued to pay my dues as we loved going to eat at the club, but having no one to play with seemed a little lonesome. I decided to take mother to ride along to play for the first time in 15 months. I had played lots of golf and many tournaments, and also played after work almost every day for years. Musgrove Golf Course was one of the most scenic in the country plus the greens were kept immaculate with bent grass. It is an 18 hole golf course with Musgrove River circling the entire course, with lots of flowers, scenic cliffs along the side and often canoes going down the river. Hole #1 was a long drive across the river, very intimidating to most people, but one of the most beautiful on this course. I told mother where to stand as I prepared to hit my first ball. I felt sure she would begin talking as she always had lots to say, but she stood there. She silently watched with lots of interest as I hit the ball and with my good luck, I hit it in a great spot over the river ready for pitching on to the green. She made mention of how far I hit the ball. I dropped my driver in my bag and off we went crossing the old fashioned swinging bridge for the next shot.

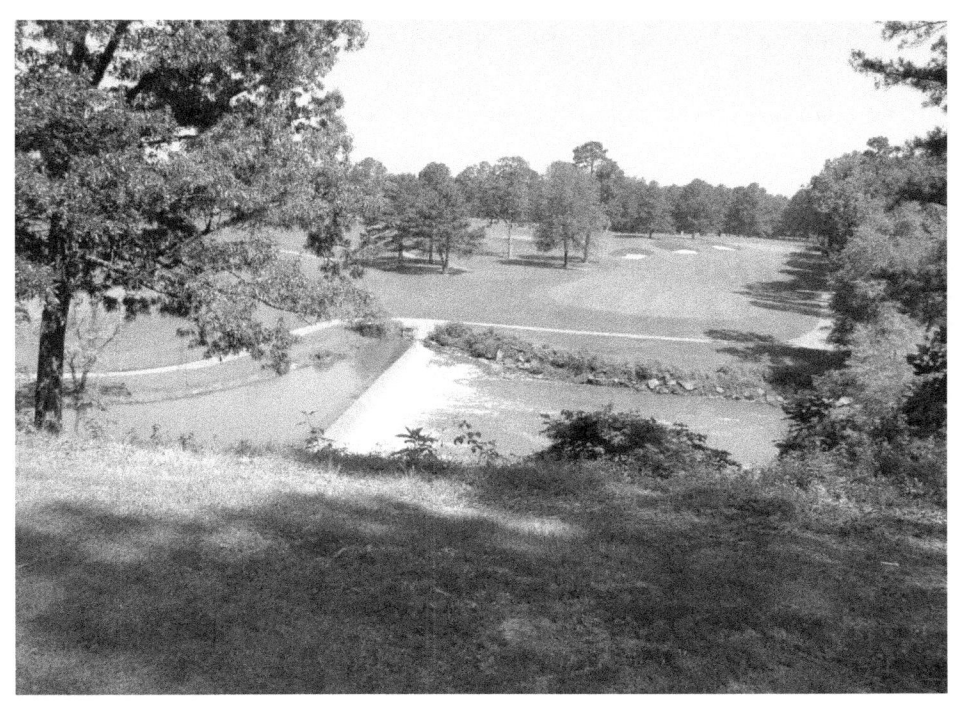

Hole #1 tees up over the Musgrove River

We were going down the steep embankment when mother began

showing the first signs of fear and did not want to ride across the

bridge. "Oh, please, Joyce Ann, let's not go across. I'm so scared we will fall in the water and it is such a far distance down there." I assured her it was safe, reached over and gently got her hand as we continued our journey for my next shot. "Mother, I began, you are always safe with me. Just hold my hand and look at the turtle down in the water. From up here you can see so many things, the beautiful rocks, little fish and sometimes an occasional ball that someone has hit the wrong way." With that she began looking for things in the water and we continued across the bridge.

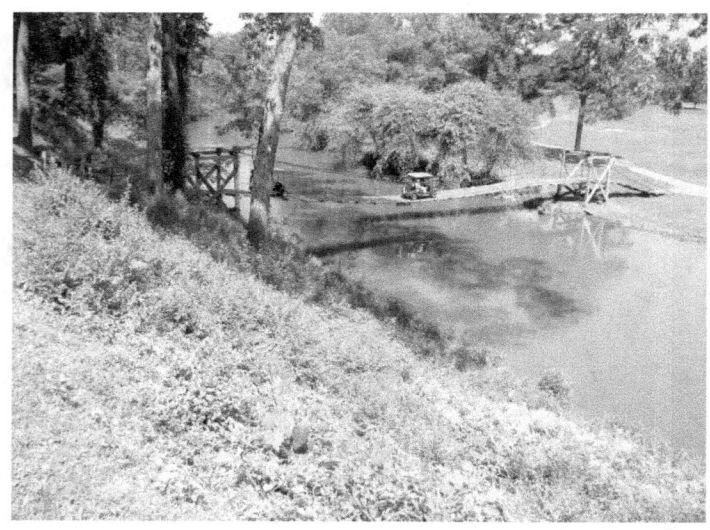

Scenic swinging bridges over the Musgrove River to the course

Once across, I stopped, got out and told her she could stand on the cart path while I hit my ball again. With that, she got out, stood beside the cart and watched again as I pitched onto the green and turned to mother explaining that she could walk to the green, but not to talk or get in front of my putt. Wow, I surprised myself with my putt. Mother laughed and clapped her hands for me, climbed back into the cart and we continued on to the next hole. She seemed to be enjoying her ride. The day was peaceful and beautiful. I teased that an angel, probably Carol, sat on my shoulder as I made that putt.

Mother loved being outside, so I knew with the day being so pretty and so many different rocks for her to look for, that she would be very content. I had also planned to get our lunch ordered and delivered out making her feel she was on a picnic. She loved picnics and made sure we enjoyed many growing up. She would plan to perfection, fry chicken golden brown, pack a big lunch in a sack as we never had a fancy picnic basket, but it was all the same to me. I knew she would also pack one of her famous big six layer chocolate cakes, which would be a high light for everyone. This day I planned to order hamburger and cokes, with cookies. I knew she would love riding and eating her lunch, listening to the birds singing, watching squirrels scampering across the path in front of us and ducks crossing the fairway. Luckily it was not a day for snakes, that is, we never saw any, but I knew they were there.

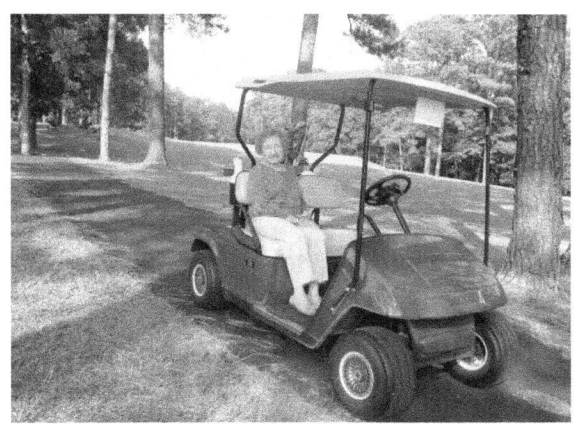

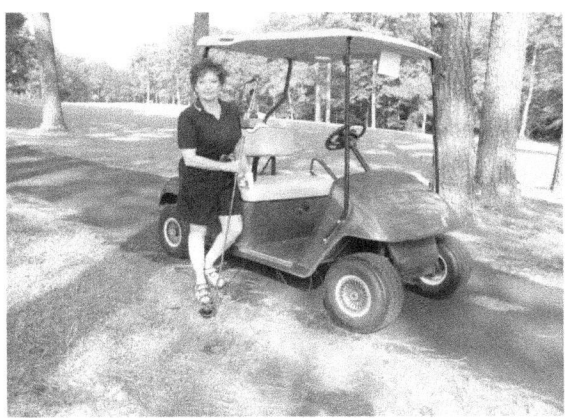

This would no doubt be a day to remember. We laughed, talked and joked as we rode the cart while she nibbled her Mr. Goodbar I had brought her as a surprise, sipping her Coke and often walking to the green while I putted.

Hole #3 was a short hole, par 3 and the shot was over a deep raven, and I was lucky again. I talked constantly to keep her attention while discussing the beauty to keep her mind off the deep raven. I said, "Now, mom I need to put this one shot across the raven and onto the green. Keep your eye on the ball for me in case I make a bad shot over into the woods or down into the raven." I hit the ball and luckily it landed on the green. She made mention again being scared to drive down the steep path, but I assured her it was safe, grabbed her hand and squeezing it gently. I smiled and said, "Oh, goodness, this is so pretty you don't have time to get scared. Let's go see where my ball is." Again, my putt was a great one and I birdied the hole telling her she was my "Good Luck Charm." She loved the compliment and we rode on knowing she was feeling important now. She loved watching the squirrels, looking for snakes, enjoyed the scenic river view and often picked up hickory nuts along the way. She picked up odd rocks and tucked them in her pockets.

While here, I remembered that Mother's love for the outdoors was dear to her heart from her life in the Mountains of Kentucky. It was all she had ever known. Her days as a child had been spent roaming the mountains with her brother, Woodrow, hunting arrow heads and appreciating God's creation of the leaves, trees, cliffs and nature, plus after she married daddy she would quickly clean house and head to the mountains to play all day. She would just get home in time to cook a hot supper for him, but sometimes she said, giggling, she would slightly burn her fried potatoes hurrying so to get his supper ready. "Oh, your dad never complained. He loved me and loved my cooking and besides he enjoyed getting home from his long day at work." She talked about her childhood and how they ate blackberries, raspberries, wild strawberries and crab apples in the summer time when they became hungry, and drank from cold spring water gushing out of the mountainside. In the fall they cracked walnuts, hickory nuts and beechnuts with rocks to satisfy their hunger pains.

It was soon time for lunch and I called in our order. "We are going to have a picnic mother, would you like that?" She smiled really big and said she would love a picnic that it had been a long time since going on one, then she began talking about how she used to plan picnics for us. The pro, Phil, brought our lunch and she was so excited to see a big hamburger with everything, French fries, coke and cookies for desert. "Don't eat your cookies yet, mom, and we will save them for a special place later to have our desert. You are going to love their hamburgers because they are known as Musgrove Burgers." She rode along, softly humming as she ate her hamburger. We stopped at Hole #15 to go to the bathroom. I had planned that half way around the course to go knowing she would hold it until we got home. "I can hold it longer than anyone," she would say, but I told her it was not healthy and we would go so we could stay out longer. She was always satisfied with answers I gave her because I tried to make her feel important and talked to her as I would my best friend, after all, she was my best friend.

Things changed when I approached the tee box on hole #15. She said, "Joyce, this is a beautiful graveyard." Startled, I turned and said, "Mother, this is a golf course, not a graveyard." "Well, look over in the distance you can see a lot of grave stones and there's a lot of people visiting their families graves. You can see the flowers they are putting on the graves." I got tickled and replied, "Mother, they are golfing just like me. This is not a graveyard." I hit the ball, not a good one and climbed back into the cart to continue my game. Again, she said, "Honey, this is the prettiest graveyard."

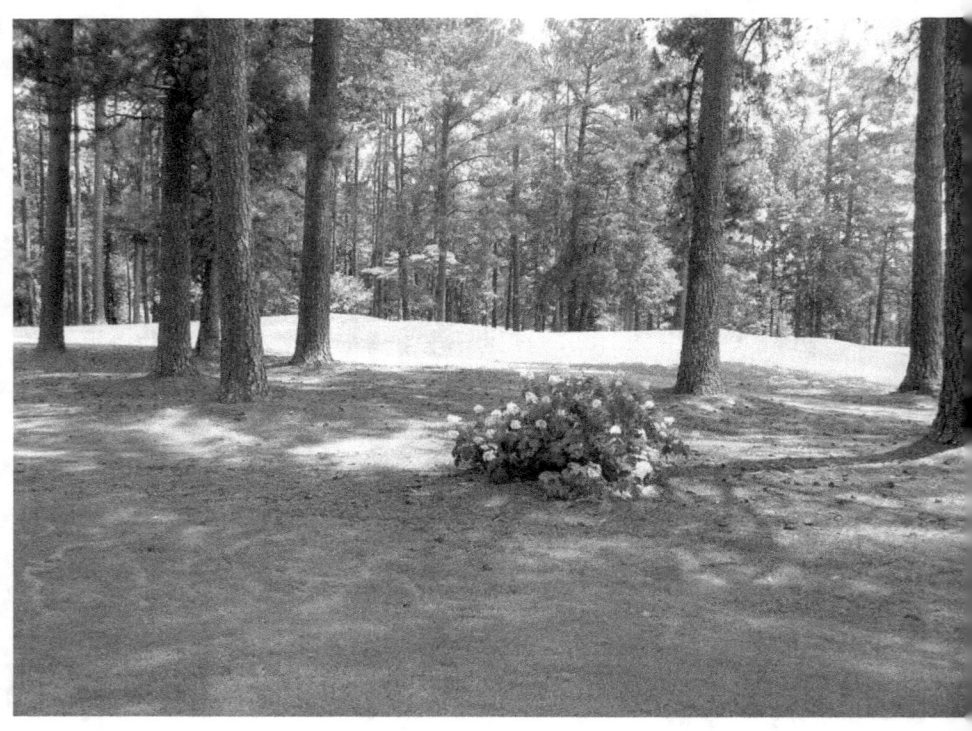

Looking back over the course, I could see how this scene could remind you of a grave?

It soon hit me that she saw the beauty of all the flowers throughout the course and thought we were playing in a graveyard. I got tickled, but had no one to share the humor with. I also tried to keep her quiet afraid someone would hear her talking about the "graveyard." By Hole #16 she was tiring and becoming confused. It had been a fun day, humorous and the birthday to remember. I finished hole #18 and we drove toward the swinging bridge to the pro shop. She looked at the river and said, "Do we have to go across that thing?" I said, "Mother, it is very strong, built with steel cable and very safe. You know I would never take you anywhere unsafe." Again, I gently reached over and took her little hand in mine, making sure she felt secure. We crossed the bridge, looked down the river and she sat back smiling knowing it was okay.

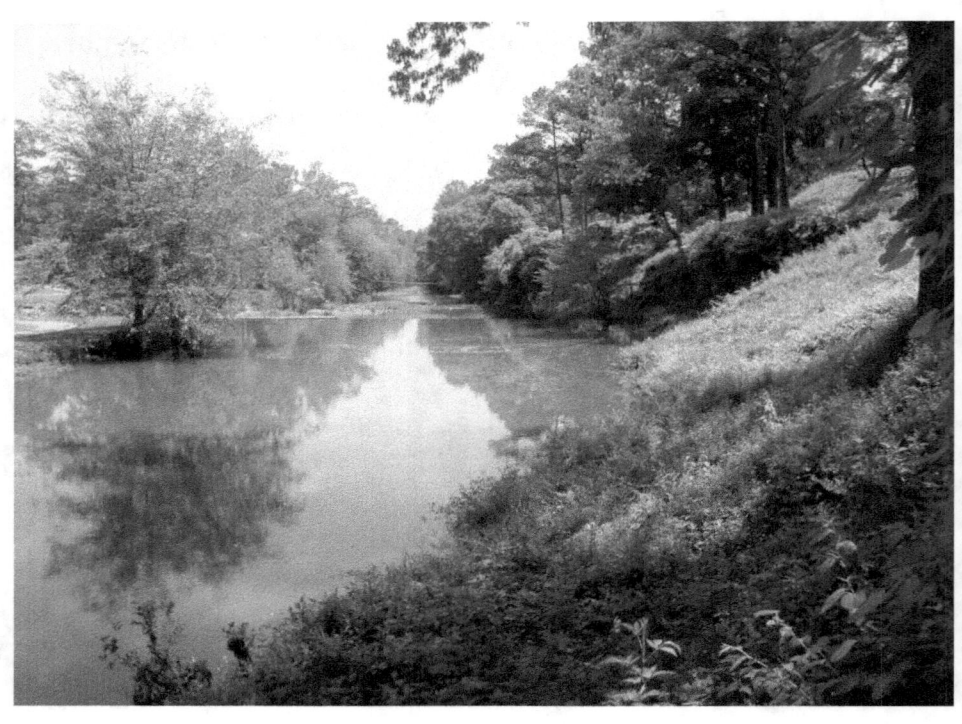

Crossing the swinging bridge from hole #18 back to the Pro Shop

I gazed off down the river, looked back at the course and wondered what the next year would bring. Would she be with me on her 88th birthday to again ride the golf cart through the graveyard? Maybe she felt the angels riding on my shoulder as I played. Yes, this would be a day to remember.

CHAPTER 16 – Putting It Bluntly

On occasions I had to take mother to my office for the day. Phyllis had an opportunity to go to Florida for a few days' vacation and my daughter and granddaughter also had to be in Florida on business for a couple of days. Their days happened to land on the same days and I had no choice but to take mother to work. She was always very patient until the late afternoon around sun downing time. At 4:00 pm she started walking the floor. I could not say I blamed her this particular day as it had been a very long one. I had tried to entertain her by putting a movie on for her to watch, giving her candy and cookies, but all this had become boring by now. She had been patient with me as she tried to kill time while I answered the phone, talked the day away of business and caught up on emails, but left her with nothing more to do than to sit and watch the TV or nap on the sofa. At home on pretty days she would walk the parking lot or walk in back of the office hunting pine cones or just wonder around. This particular day it was raining buckets of water and she could not go out.

At noon I asked if she was hungry. Eating out was a favorite and of course she said she was very hungry. We soon left for the mall grabbing chicken nuggets at Chic Fil-A. We killed some time walking through Belk's and climbed back into the car to run by my daughter's house to check on her pit bulls that were due to have puppies. "Mother," I began, "I have to run by Kim's to check on her dogs." "How many does she have," she asked. "Mother, it is Kim's dogs next door. Remember she has three and two are due to have puppies. You just have that a little wrong," she cut in and said to me, "I know, Joyce Ann, short term memory." I screamed with laughter and we both laughed hard. I said, "Mother, you truly amaze me." She went on, "Well, that's what you always say, so I just beat you to it."

Sometimes I wondered just how much those with dementia really do understand and comprehend, but say nothing. Mother had always been witty and quick thinking. I often had twinges of hurt thinking about how she was caged into this new world that she did not understand. She had always had freedom in those beautiful mountains of Kentucky, now we lived in an area that would not allow her to walk through those sacred woods, sit on rocks and gaze out over the valley below. She no longer had the freedom to drive to the Cumberland River and skip rocks across the water. Her freedom now relied within the dependence on me to support all her needs. She was quick to tell me how much she loved me and appreciated me. She often reminded me that she was a burden, which broke my heart to hear her say the words that she really felt. When I tucked her to bed at night she would reach up and gently pull my face me down to her. I looked down into those sparkling hazel eyes always with a big beautiful smile gracing her face, and she would place a kiss goodnight on my forehead before she snuggled down between the sheets. She thanked me often for everything I did for her. I could tell she was getting slower daily. She now walked behind me instead of with me. She took longer to put her feet into the pants leg I held for her as I dressed her. While I cooked, she was often behind me and sometimes as I stepped backward I would walk back into her, so close as if she felt I too would suddenly be gone, but then she would laugh and say, "I'm sorry, honey. I didn't mean to be in your way." She no longer pin curled her hair or applied makeup. I pin curled her hair sometimes before she went to bed. It was all in my daily routine to make sure she felt good and was safe.

It takes patience and understanding to deal with dementia, but those with patience and giving love will soon understand it is all about feeling insecure. With lots of patience and love, they will feel secure. It was a daily reassurance to be with them when they went to bed, and important to turn out their lights, tuck them into their bed and explain that all is well within the house. I would now close the door to mother's bedroom and she loved sleeping in a dark room with the door closed. I had come to realize that when I closed the door, she never got back up, but if she closed the door she had a hard time settling down. When I realized the difference, I soon realized she felt secure when I closed her door while she was safely in bed. I also began to put my hands gently over her eyes and tell her to close her beautiful hazel eyes and go to sleep and she soon went to sleep very quickly. She knew I would be there with her for any needs she may have. Simple things made such a big difference. All was well within the house when mother was in bed, but I still could not find those girdles!

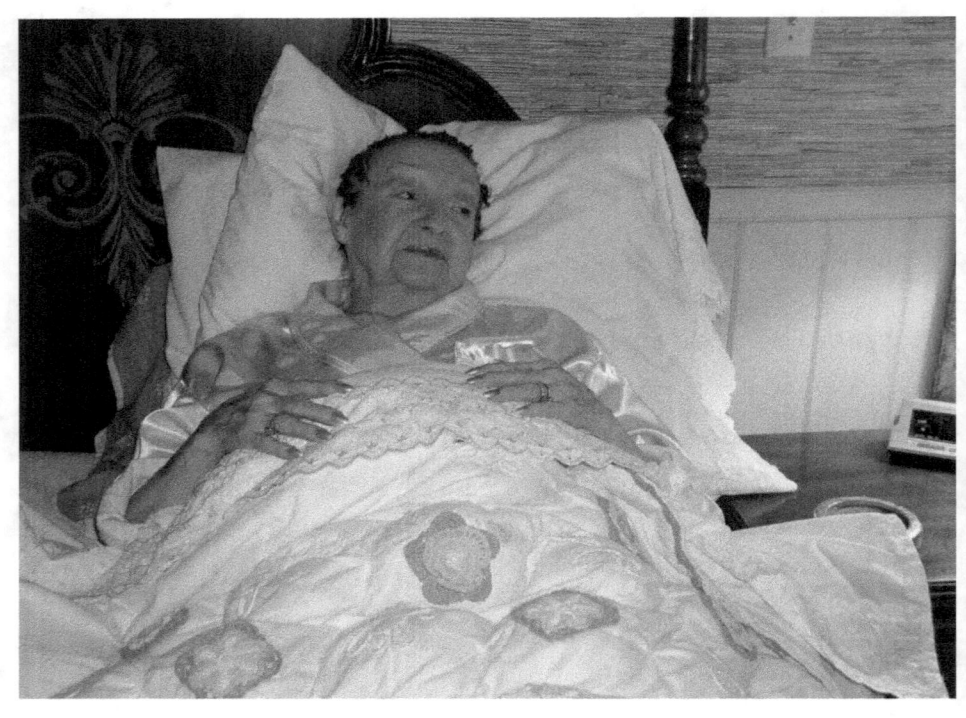

Mother all tucked in bed with her hair pin curled.

CHAPTER 17 – Christmas 2006

With each season brought new experiences with mother. I noticed she would get a bit annoyed when company came if it was people she was not familiar with. Even my daughter and granddaughter, who lived next door, made her irritable at times. This was a part of the illness I could not understand. It could be she felt that they were invading her home, or she may have felt they were taking me away from her time. Mother was very demanding when it came to attention. It seemed to be the threesome that made her uncomfortable. When she was in those moods I tried harder to give her more attention. It may or may not help depending on her mood for the given day. With the extra chores it made mother a real handful to watch. She did not want to go to Kim's, but with a little encouraging and telling her I needed her help, instead of demanding she go with me, always proved to be successful. It was a feeling I thought about myself not wanting to do something someone else did, so I knew she may not always be in favor of doing what I wanted her to do. If I negotiated with her, or made her feel she was needed, it would soon win her over my way.

Kim had two sets of puppies due and I was one happy camper when she got back from her trip. The puppies finally arrived. Both the mothers came in within a day of each other and sixteen, beautiful, healthy puppies arrived. I knew that if Kim asked me to babysit the puppies that there was no way I could have taken care of sixteen puppies, mother and the office. When they were four weeks old they had their first outing. I took mother over to Kim's and watched as she unloaded all sixteen squirmy, barking puppies out of their boxes and into the yard. What a sight. Mother loved babies and animals. This was "her" day for sure. Kim picked up one of the puppies and said, "Here Grandma, hold this baby." Mother cuddled the puppy into her arms and I watched as she enjoyed the sweetness of this little guy snuggling into the warmth of her neck. She smiled like a child. Christmas would soon be here and she knew some child would own one of these new baby puppies. I knew I could not give one to mother, but she did have our cat Shadow. She was definitely enough to take care for and to have two babies would be too much. I could see the gleam in her eyes as she cuddled and nurtured the new baby. I also knew they had bonded. For some reason, old people and cats or puppies just go together. At least we were next door so she could continue to enjoy all the new babies until they found homes.

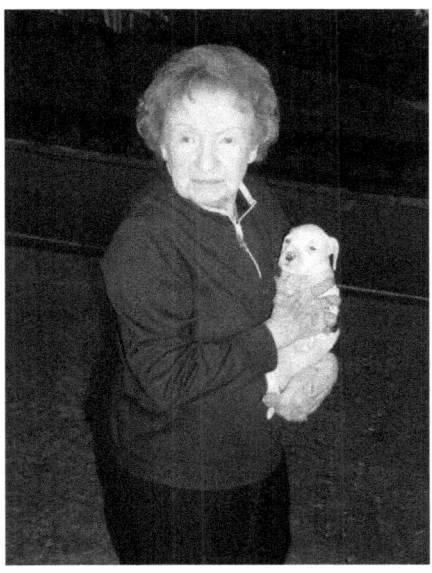

Mother with the new 4 week old pit bull puppy and did not want to give him up

After we left Kim's we walked back to the house talking about the sweet little cuddles. We shopped earlier in the day and had lots of Christmas gifts to wrap. I pulled all of last years wrapping paper out of the basement, along with the bows, name tags and tape. I sat down in the center of the great room and began wrapping, carefully placing the items close to me for safe keeping. Mother first took a notice to the the scissors while I was stirring the spaghetti on the stove. These scissors took time to find. Next she took my sweater off the chair and with much haste she took off to her bedroom. With her pace you would have thought a fire had erupted in the house. You would also think after chasing her four times down the hall I would know better. I next missed the name tags. She had somehow taken them while I obviously had my back turned for no more than one moment. Oh, Lord, how fast this lady traveled. I found the name tags on the side table next to where she was sitting. "Oh my," I thought, "how could I get dinner ready, wrap gifts and know where mother was every minute. Not to mention trying to keep up with all the things I needed to finish this project. At long last, I wrapped all the gifts for the evening, hid the paper in the closet and thought to myself, out of sight, out of mind. With mother, if it was in sight it was "gone." It could be very easy to become an alcoholic when you have to deal with this, but thanks to God, inner strength kept me going. I did have a beer in the evenings to take the edge off. Between the two I prevailed.

Mornings were always the same. I tried to watch her door for the first crack of light seeping out from around the door. If I caught her in time I could get her in the shower, but if not, it was another confrontation for the beginning of a new day. This always tired me and often I did the spot wash instead of trying to totally undress her to get her into the shower. She would always assure me that she had her bath, had clean clothes on and had brushed her teeth.

Mother would definitely put you on the defensive and it kept me on my toes to stay ahead of her. She was quiet as a mouse, could walk through the house in shoes made of cotton. She floated as if on clouds making it harder to know where she was. The house was a good sized house, all one level, and designed so you could actually walk a circle. This also posed a problem. Sometimes when I went hunting for her, she had taken the opposite route and I ended up walking the circle trying to catch up with her. A comical view if one could see, but a frustrating situation when I could not find her. Sometimes she just would not answer when I called. It was almost like she played head games with me and I think she did. She had always been one to play practical jokes, loved to laugh and often played jokes on my father. Once when he came in from the mines, all black with coal dust, she had his bath water ready in the big tub she had fixed in the back of the house. As she recalled, "I told your dad his bath water was ready and to go ahead and get in." I watched him and told my brother Murphy what I was going to do. He said, "Emily, Calvin will kill you." "Aw," she told him, "It's all in fun." Once he had lathered up with the Lifebuoy Soap, had his face all covered in suds, she slipped and set off a pack of firecrackers. This was during the mining problems and she said daddy came jumping out of the tub trying to get to his gun. Of course mother had a good laugh with her brother. I am sure my daddy did not think it was too funny.

The weeks had flown by that year and here it was three weeks before Christmas. It was a usual Sunday morning as I tiptoed to her bedroom and could see light through the crack under her door, so I knew she was alive and up. When I entered her bedroom, I noticed she had already made her bed and was also out of her pajamas. "Mother, "I began, "I don't want you to get dressed just yet. We have to wash our hair this morning. It is Sunday and I want you to wear that beautiful new Christmas sweater Phyllis bought you."

"I have clean clothes on, Joyce, and I like what I have picked out to wear today." I go to the closet, bring out the new sweater and continue, "Mother, look how pretty this is. It is much prettier than what you have, plus it is new." She stands looking at the sweater, studying the situation and then continued, "Well, I guess it is nicer. So I will wear that instead of this, but I will wear this one tomorrow." With that I coaxed her to come to the kitchen while I popped a couple of biscuits in the oven.

"Mother, do you want jelly and biscuits or honey and biscuits," I asked? "I would rather have honey and biscuits". My Dad always said honey was good for you and he had bee hives so he knew all about bees and honey. Why he used to have Mom wrap him up, tie his clothes to his wrists and ankles and he could rob the bee hives. I loved her stories, maybe over and over, but they never got old to me. I knew each and every one would be passed on to my children and grandchildren. She continued, "We stood and watched him

from the window and my Dad never got stung one single time."
With that she was happy and ready for her honey and biscuits.

"Let's go to the office and let me check my emails while the biscuits are baking." Off we go, with her trailing behind me, to my office just opposite of the kitchen. Sundays were easier than Saturday. Mother loved preaching and singing. I would tune in a good spiritual program that had great religious music and she would stay indefinitely. Mother knew her bible. She often spoke the phrases or recited the verses along with the minister. She would also sing along with songs she knew, "Oh Happy Day, Oh Happy Day, or Always on the Sunny Side, Always on the Sunny Side." Many times she would continue singing these throughout the day, which amazed me to hear her remember those wonderful old songs.

She sang Jingle Bells a lot and I could tell she realized Christmas was near. Mother had been a very seasonal person; made sure every holiday was special and planned Christmas all year to make sure this was the most special day of the year. She hid change throughout the year to save to buy her gifts. And from doilies and under rugs she would gather her saved money, making her lists and making sure everyone got a gift. We had very little growing up as my father was so sick most of my life with the Black Lung, but mother kept our household together, with lots of love and reassurance that all was well, even as I look back and remember times when all was not well. I knew with the thoughts I could see in her mind I would have to watch all the gifts now lying under the tree. Without eyes in both the front and back of my head, Mother would have all these gifts tucked neatly into her bedroom, oh, mind you, for safe keeping. This year I had bought Christie Karaoke. It was heavy and to lug that thing to her bedroom would have been an ordeal. I am sure she had the given that big gift much thought.

What thoughts they have, how does their brain function, shifting from moment to moment and they can rattle your cage more than the worst earthquake. If you learn patience and endurance you get through the rough days, but remember when they were the parent you were the child. How she chased me when I was a child, could not keep up with me because I was a very busy child but she made sure I was bathed at night even when I fussed I was too tired from my day of playing to take my bath. We learn to give back what we had been given. My, but I wonder where those darned girdles could be hidden. Sometimes I would lie at night screening every inch of that house trying to think of where they could be, but oh, well, I am sure they will surface one day. Along with the girdles were now stashed the pictures I had printed that were lying on top of the new frames I bought to give to her grandchildren for Christmas. These may show up next year, but it had been a year and still no sign of the girdles. When I faced these obstacles with mother I had to realize that I too could be walking in her shoes one day.

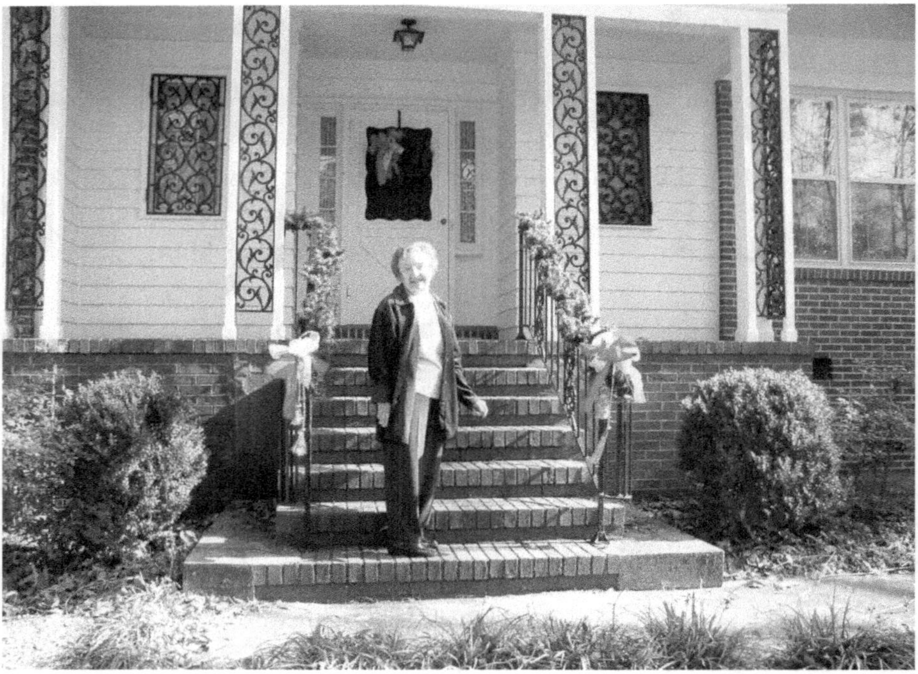

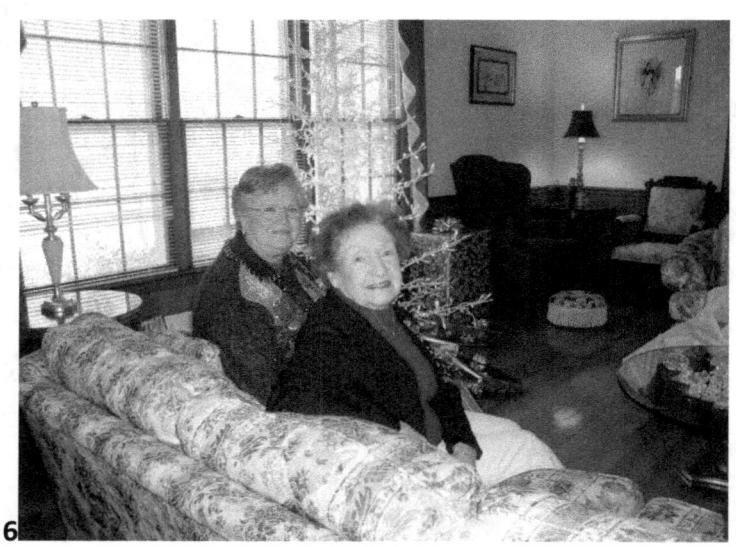

Mother loves Christmas and having her picture taken (Dec. 2006)

Mother and Phyllis - Christmas 2006

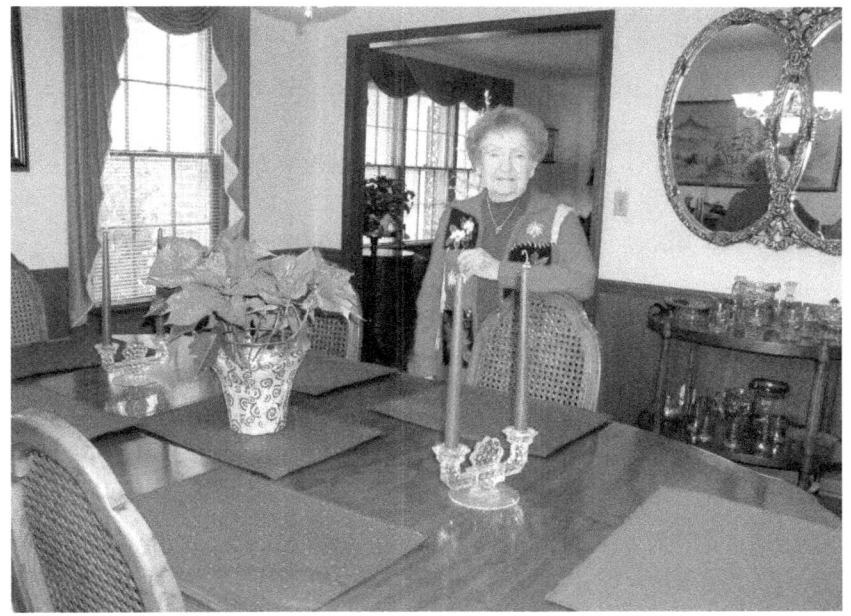

CHAPTER 18 – Moments to Remember

Looking back it seems only yesterday that I was the child, she was the mother. I knew that one day she would be floating out there watching out for me again. Her spirit would be strong as she was a strong woman. I knew she would always be there as she had always been there for me. Mothers are very special people. They cared for you when you felt no one else cared. They protected you when no one else would protect you. They would give you their last penny to make you happy when no one else helped. They noticed when your heart was heavy, when no one else cared if it broke and they would be missed forever.

My mother, was also raised in a loving family, but I cannot recall anyone having dementia and Alzheimer's was unheard of back then. I remember some were said to have "gone lost their mind," but it was called the old age disease. Her family was very poor, but their hearts were very rich. She was the runt of sixteen children.

The first born daughter had tragically died a horrible death after lighting her toy corncob pipe in the fireplace as her parents and grandparents slept and catching her night gown on fire. Her parents would have seven boys before having another girl. Mother weighed in at 2 ½ lbs and had pneumonia at three months old and came into the world fighting. She slept in a dresser drawer on a pillow. Because of her small size she would not have the honor of attending school until she was eight years old. She learned at an early age to work in the gardens, cook and help with the chores. Her brothers adored her. She would marry and birth three girls, only to lose her youngest to the hands of a foster child. It would be the tragedy that sent her into orbit, to a zone where she would never return, one that I would never forget, but even when she knew she was not well, she still fought a hard fight to hold her own. She was quick to tell you that she had stored things in the back of her head, as she pointed where these were and where she would no longer go and cut you off if you suggested looking at family photos. "I'm not ready to look at those, Joyce Ann," she would say and I would not push her. Sometimes I tried gently hoping it would bring her back to me, but after many months and years I knew she would never be the same.

It had been almost seven years since that horrible year of losing five of her loved ones, but she would tell you in a heartbeat that she was not ready to talk about it and the subject would always drop. "Oh, later," Joyce Ann," she would say, "but I am not ready to go back there just yet."   I wondered if she was shutting out part of her world so she would not have to think about it again, whether she wanted to go there, but knew it would not be a good thing to attempt, and I never pushed her in any way. I am sure in her own way she felt safe with not thinking back. Oh, she would talk about her mom and dad and often stand at their pictures in the hall and tell them how much she loved them. She would never go back to her daughter Carol.

Mother spent her life providing for her family. It was all she would ever know. If you said, "You have never worked." She got angry, making her feel intimidated and would tell you how she had spent her days picking beans in the garden and half the night cleaning and breaking them to prepare for the winters food supply. She made sure her buttermilk biscuits were just the right shade of brown before taking them out of the coal burning oven. Mornings were spent frying eggs, bacon, ham, sausage and making gravy to go with her hot biscuits. Jugs of honey and sorghum syrup with ladles sat in the middle of the table. We would eat as a family and hold hands for thanking God for what we had. We were taught to care for each other.

I watched as she continued to live in the past, which I felt was good at times. We never went to bed without family prayer. It would be mother that led the pathway to church and it was mother that held the family together. She still prayed her prayers, beautiful prayers, but she no longer read her bible. Those were some of the things I would never understand, but I felt I had found just the right button to always get through to her and to guide her when she wanted or pulled a different way.

When mother's mother was diagnosed with cancer of the uterus, it was mother that took care of her and she carried hot meals to her dad every single day until his death. When her dad was lost in the Mountains of Kentucky, it was mother that took him to her home and cared for him and when he was hit with a car one evening as she let him get out at the church, it was mother that cared for him until his death. She never gave a second thought to not being there for the family in times of need. For me, it was not a sacrifice to care for her, it was what was expected of me to do. It was my job, my pay back for all the caring she had given to me and others. I never resented this care and it was a joy to always see her smiling face knowing she was happy with me.

My father called her pint sized and teased about how tough she was to be so little. She carried herself like a movie star and worked like a lumberjack. She could work until sweat poured off her, and her clothes soaking wet, but she was both sexy and tough.

If she was confronted with problems, she attacked it with a vengeance, but listened to reasoning. We dared not cross her and knew she carried a heavy blow with her hands if we disobeyed.

Mother was one of the wittiest of anyone I had ever known. I never knew what was coming out of her mouth next, but she loved to laugh. She was creative and I often wondered what she could have become

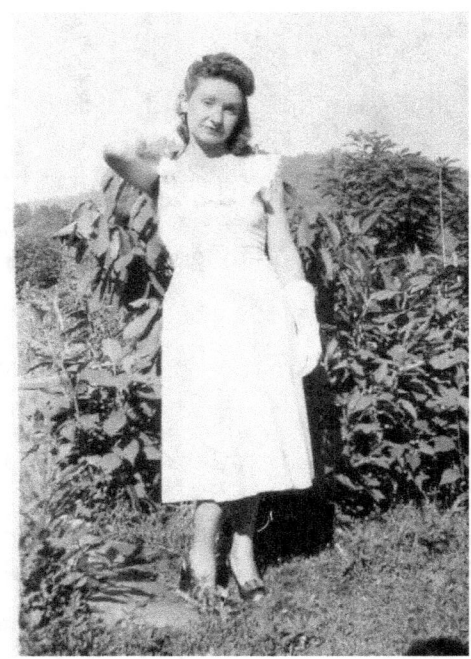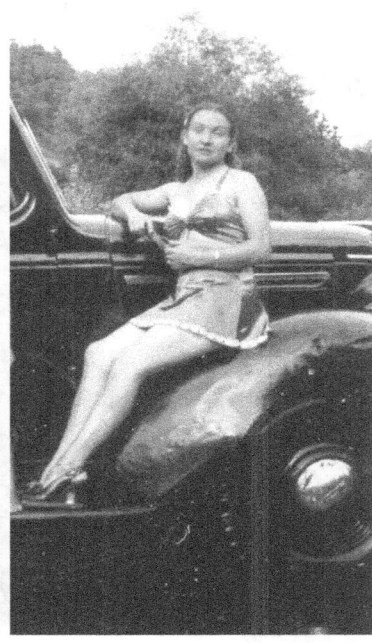

Mother at 24 years old

if given the opportunity. She was a marvelous decorator. Her

creations were limitless. We were raised with a budget, well, more

like pennies and had to make every penny count. She changed the

house every spring, making a new little castle from her creative

mind.

Mother was very creative and even with the dementia she still rearranged our furniture when I least expected a change. I remember when she took an old lanoline rug, painted it white with high gloss enamel, cut sponges into diamonds, squares and dipped the sponge in red and black high gloss enamel. She first used a ruler to make a perfect black border, leaving the center of the rug white. Next, she dipped the diamond sponge into the black paint and the square into red paint. She alternated the design, let the rug dry and placed it in the center of the kitten. Next she painted the old chairs high gloss white enamel. The little table was white with a thin red line design around the top, with the side's red. When my father came in from work he could not believe this beautiful new kitchen. She also had a hot supper on the stove with hot cornbread waiting to come out of the oven. On the sideboard in the dining room she had baked a chocolate pie, a coconut pie and butterscotch pie. The three pies made it hard to eat our supper, but we knew we had to eat properly or we would not have desert.

Now she was still creative with her jewelry and her clothes as she put on several rings, loved shiny things and enjoyed dressing up. She would rearrange the pillows on the sofa, or move a chair, but in her little twisted mind, I could still see her vision from times past, still trying to be functional, but somehow things did not go together for her.

My memories as a child were of wonderful aromas as I entered our front door, enjoying the beauty of a sparkling home and knowing we would sleep in clean smelling sheets that had dried from the clothes line in the back yard. I never worried about anything when I went to sleep and had fond memories as I was awakened in the mornings to the smell of hot coffee, hot chocolate and bacon frying. Mother was gentle with getting us out of bed. She always planted a tender kiss on our forehead and gently told us it was time to get up. She also asked what we wanted for breakfast, giving us choices of eggs, biscuits, cream o' wheat, oatmeal, sugared toast, milk toast or French toast. It never bothered her to prepare everyone a different breakfast. Her interest was making sure we had a healthy hot breakfast to start our day.

Yes, memories of my mother's caring would go on forever. I never felt I had to worry about her love for me, but now it was my turn to make sure she received the same from me in her last days. I felt one of the lucky ones with mother's dementia progressing very slowly. She never went into the fetal position, passed the aggressive stage, continued to be active and sometimes too active, but for me it continued to be a challenge daily.

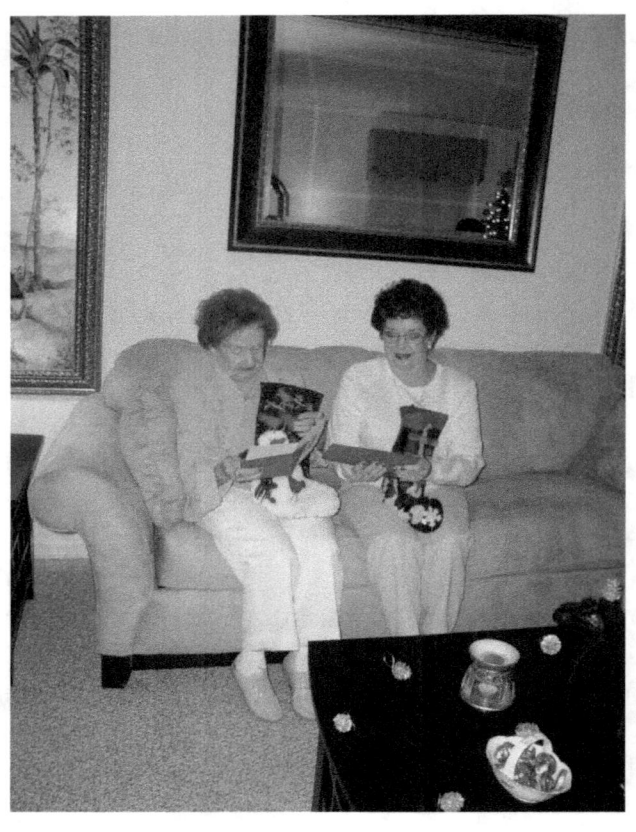

Enjoying Christmas at Kim's with her very own Christmas stocking Kim gave her. Mother was now Kim's child also. We gave her lots of love and attention. Yes, mother was easy to love. (Dec. 2007)

CHAPTER 19 – Good Morning Baby Pollywog

"Good morning little Pollywog.

How can you see in such a fog?

To swim around from log to log,

You little baby Pollywog…………

It was December 21, 2006 when she came into my office singing Little Baby Pollywog. I had never heard the song before and as she laughed, with the twinkle in her hazel blue eyes, she stopped at my desk and shook her little finger delightfully singing and acting out the song. Most of the time she sang "Yankee Doodle," but I knew when mother was singing she was happy and I also knew she felt secure. She was confident. She was a joy. You might ask if I missed having a friend, a date for dinner once in a while or my freedom. I would answer, yes, but I would miss mother more. It made my heart skip beats of love for her as I watched this little lady move to her own music. She had always been dramatic singing to us when we were a child and acting out her songs. I remember how she belted out "John Henry was a steel driving man sitting on his pappy's knee," as she would pound her knees and then sing "Oh My Darling, Oh My Darling, Oh My Darling Clementine." We were loved. We felt secure. We felt confident. We were her joy.

I remember when I had to move her out of her beautiful home high in the mountains of Harlan, Kentucky. It was a night to remember plus a livid nightmare. While going through the house I found beautiful cashmere hats from Paris that had been left to mother from a great aunt. I put one on her and tucked one on me and began doing the Charleston. Wow, I could not believe she followed the dance, kicking up her heels and we laughed, sang and danced until we could hardly breathe. It was a memorable moment forever engraved in my mind laughing harder than we could talk. Oh, did I have fun with my sweet mother.

This particular Christmas would be special and a day to be remembered. Kim had baked the turkey; I made the special cornbread dressing I learned from mother, flavored heavy with sage. Christie invited her new special friend, and we celebrated with a bottle of Asti Spumante. Mother enjoyed a "sip" and toasted as we all laughed. We had our usual circle of prayer with each contributing to their special thanks to God for this wonderful day. I led prayer and was thankful for having my family with me and we passed on to the next person to give their special thanks to God. Mother followed thanking God for the food and our family and friends. Kim was next as she was the eldest daughter, thanking God for letting them live next door and providing them with their needs. Christie thanked God for her special family and asked God to let her find her brother. Greg thanked God for allowing him to be a part of this special family. None had a dry eye as we all said together, "Amen." We were a very loving, caring family and the spirit in our home was one a stranger could feel, soft, humble and knowing it was filled with God's presence, as well as my mother's. Everyone watched Mother as she proceeded to put her cranberry sauce on top of her macaroni and cheese, never batting an eye and began eating as if all was well. We all looked at each other, raising an eyebrow and then we all burst out laughing so hard, but she missed the joke, but she joined in the laughter always making sure she was part of the party. Yes, it was a special Christmas and I sat looking at her, wondering if she would be with us next year. We all dug into the turkey, dressing, macaroni and cheese, mashed potatoes, giblet gravy, deviled eggs, congealed salad, sweet potato soufflé, baked beans and rolls. Phyllis made Pecan Pie, Banana Nut Bread and Chocolate Cake. Kim brought fresh baked cookies. It was a fun day. As I looked at mother I thought about the girdles still missing, now adding to the list were her leather coat and new Christmas sweater that Phyllis had given her. Oh, what a day and what a special little lady, but it was all worth it.

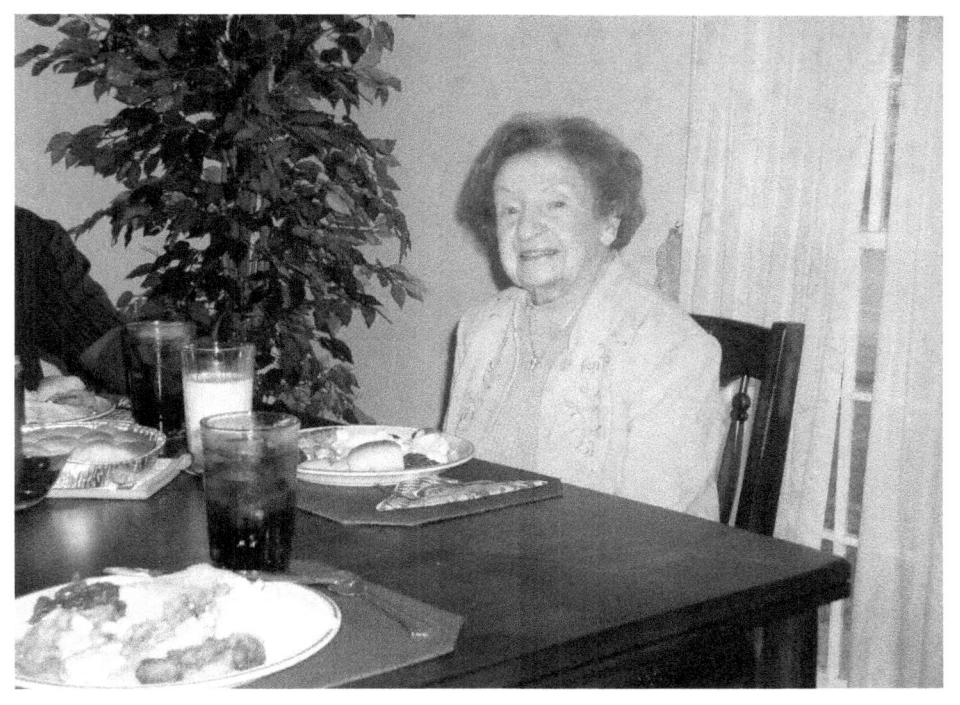

Emily, Christmas dinner at Kim's 2006

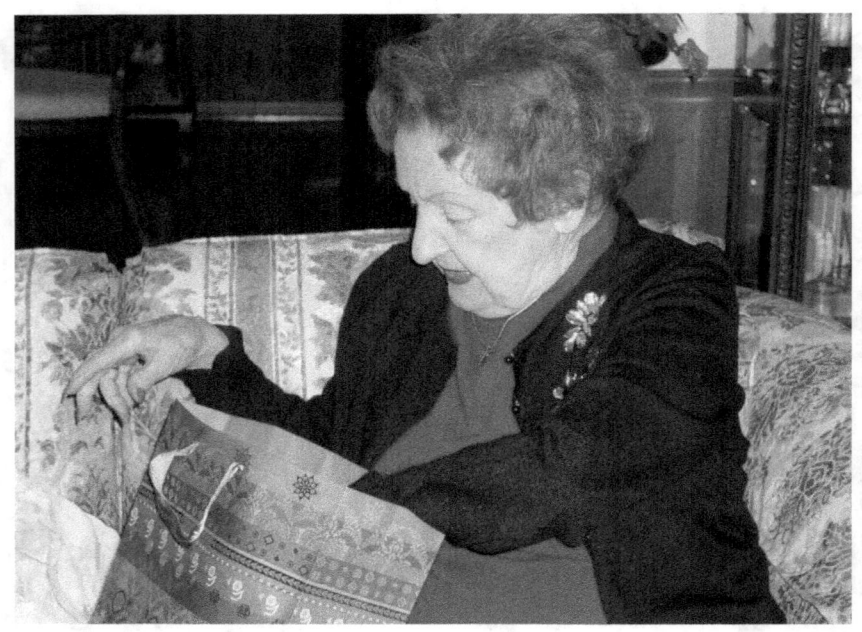

Mother loved gifts...............

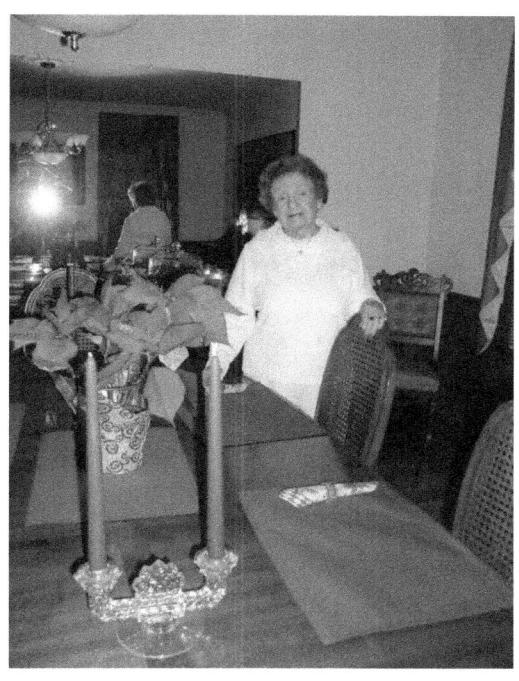

Mother wearing her now missing sweater. It, no doubt, was safely tucked away along with the leather coat, girdles, socks, and other items that would hopefully surface "one" day in some strange place.

Mother thought about others, putting them first ahead of everything. Years ago when my stepfather came down with the flu she worried about his depression. He had been bedridden for two weeks. One morning she slipped into one of the bedrooms, hunted out an old blond wig with long hair. She then found a bright red sultry shorty sheer nightie. Next, she found a pair of very bright red spiked heels. She also came across a pair of black mesh hose. Her outfit was almost complete except she decided to put on white lace gloves up to the elbow, bright red lipstick and found a "fancy" purse. With that she put her new outfit on, yelled down the hall and said, "Frank, are you dressed?" He said, "Well yes, honey I am." She said, "Frank, are you sure you are dressed? We have a visitor." With that, he called back, "Yes, Emily, I am dressed." She then went into a very sexy routine, dancing into his bedroom, twirling her purse around in circles, singing a stripper's song, kicking her heels high in the air like a Rockette and making a dramatic entrance. She stopped as she slung one glove off, turned her back to Frank, and wiggled her butt as she pulled the other glove off. With that she said dad came jumping out of bed and started laughing and kissing her. I am sure this was not all to the story, as she held back laughing with a little twinkle in her eyes, and a shade red to her cheeks. She did say he recovered quickly from his depression and flu.

Mother was also very witty and loved laughing. My stepfather explained, "I had a big pimple on my nose and your mother said she would fix it. She did. She put some kind of ointment on my nose. I was allergic to whatever she used and my nose swelled so big, my glasses would not fit and my eyes nearly swelled together. I could not go to church to preach that Sunday. She laughed so hard she cried." With that, mother began laughed again as I reminded her of the story. I found it strange that she always remembered some of those stories from her past in such detail. My dad went on, "Your mom did not do it once, but she did it twice," he continued as he held up two fingers, smiling with a twinkle in his eyes. "It took a whole week for my nose to get back to normal so I could wear my glasses." We all screamed with laughter.

Yes, she will be remembered and one day I will find the girdles, leather coat, socks, panties, and will be surprised with what else could be hidden in the enclosure of our home. I am sure when these items surface my feelings will be mixed with laughter and tears thinking about this little lady who was my mother. She loved

life and loved the outdoors, but she loved God and her family more.

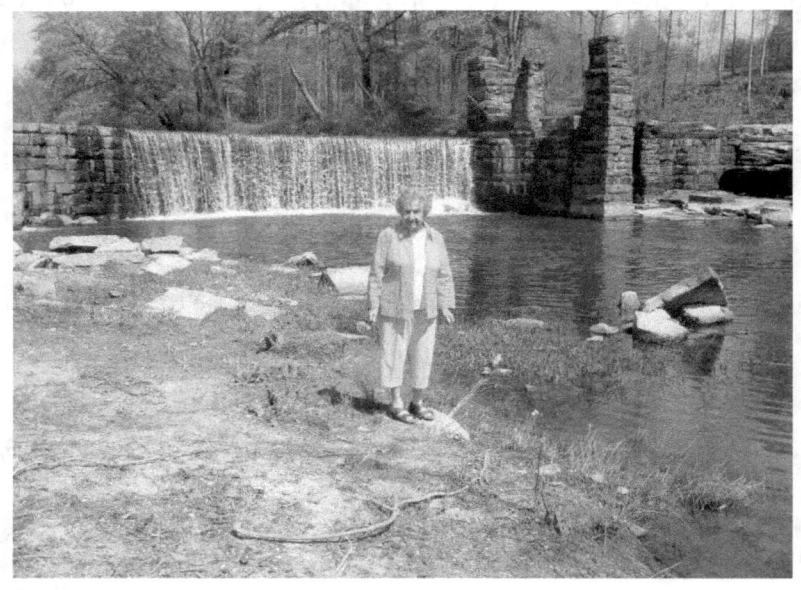

A Sunday outing at the Old Mill in Townley, AL – March, 2007

CHAPTER 20 - Panic Attack – My Diamond

It had been months since Christmas and finally the beautiful sweater lost since Christmas was found by Kim while hunting in my office for business papers. Kim found the sweater all neatly folded in one of my desk drawers tucked in between the Pendaflex files. The leather coat was finally found behind a chair in the sun room. It is no longer a shock to find missing items months later.

It was one of those rare times that I got sick, but it happened. I had spent the weekend dozing and trying to keep my eyes on mother. She was definitely regressing. That night I placed all my jewelry in the usual place on my dresser. My special diamond necklace was carefully laid out, next to the jewelry box for my rings. I hardly remembered taking it off my neck. The weekend was mostly a blur, trying to fight not sleeping and too sick to get up and hunt for mother in the other room. I had pneumonia again and could hardly think straight as all I wanted to do was to just lie in bed. At times I thought she was in her bedroom sorting out her drawers or combing her hair. I knew she was safe and felt no threat of her leaving because it was cold and rainy.

Monday morning I showered, got mother showered and dressed and when I went to my dresser to put on my jewelry, to my horror, the diamond necklace was gone. I totally panicked, frantically looking behind the dresser to see if it could have been knocked off the dresser during the night. This was a special gift from Ed and now being a widow; it was like a dagger stabbing me in the chest. I panicked, and called Kim as I continued my search.

By the time Kim came over, Phyllis had arrived to care for mother for the day and we all began hunting. It was fruitless. This diamond was the most expensive piece of jewelry I owned. It was a beautiful, rare, German cut trillion solitaire and was given to me on Valentine's Day many years ago. I cried hard, but no diamond. I prayed and tried to think where mother could have hid the diamond. She loved jewelry and anything that sparkled. We continued the search. I would come home during the day, while Phyllis had mother out, searching for my diamond. It was hard to keep my mind on my business and my tears would not stop flowing. Kim also searched the house while no one was home, but no diamond.

Two months had passed and no sign of the diamond. We all knew it was in the house, but like the sweater thinking she had hid it in one of the bedrooms, we were surprised to find it in my office. The diamond was probably wrapped in a napkin or handkerchief and tucked into a "safe" secure place. She wrapped coins, buttons and small items, neatly finding secure, safe places for keeping. I should have known better as I had watched other things disappear. I was so worried that it caused a peak in my already problem blood pressure. During that time I had to have tests thinking I had heart blockage, but no doubt it was stress from the strain of losing my diamond. How silly of me to be so attached to something, but I could not help my feelings. The tears dried, my blood pressure came down and I had to come to terms with myself that I would find the diamond one day. No, I could not get mad with mother. She never knew what was going on. She tried to hunt, but as I watched her I knew she had no earthly idea what she was looking for. How could you blame someone that no longer functioned normally? It was actually my very own fault. Kim had warned me many times that I should be locking my bedroom door, which I did have a lock put on, but had become a little careless with my personal belongings. Mother followed me trying to help in the hunt, but did not realize what she was hunting. I had to also stop hunting while she was home. She hunted desperately, but could not understand what she was looking for. I could tell it was making her very nervous. It soon became clear the stress was too much for her and only continued my search during times she was away from the house.

I again realized the diamond was like the girdles, which have never been found. Nor the many things too numerous to count, but one day, I am sure I would find that little hole in the wall where mother found a special place to tuck away her treasures. Funny, how the missing white Christmas sweater reappeared. Yes, Mother got up one morning wearing the white sweater!

It would be nine months before the diamond actually "reappeared!" Each night I helped mother get ready for bed, picking out a nice gown or pj's, helping her empty her pockets and tucking her safely in and kissing her goodnight. This would be a different night. She was happy and had her pockets full of "junk." I held my hands out together and said, "Put your goodies in my hands and I will put them in your tray until morning." She reached into her right pocket and as she unloaded her things, I noticed a sparkle from the overhead light catching my eye. As I turned around I looked closely and there in my hands, among all her marbles, buttons and a few other treasures, lay my diamond necklace. I quickly picked it out and stuck it in my pocket. That was a happy night for me. As I turned to mother, I smiled and said, "You had some real goodies in there tonight mom." She laughed and said she saved everything she found. I could not believe the diamond reappeared in her pants pocket after nine long months, but as I walked out her bedroom door I was thanking God for answering my many prayers.

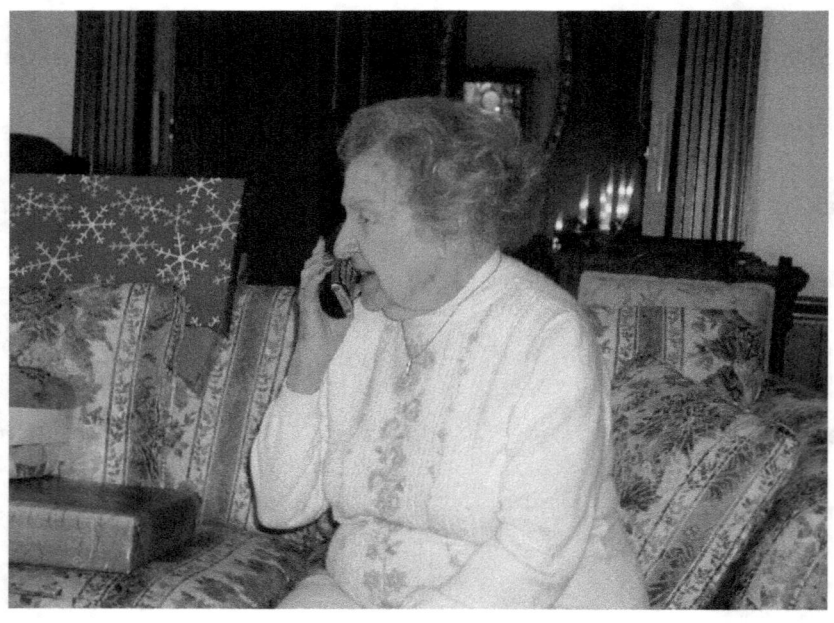

Mother was always happy and loved talking on the phone, sometimes picking it up up-side-down

CHAPTER 21 - The Dark Side

August 6, 2007 was the day from hell. The news was blunt, not news I was prepared to hear, but in the back of my mind I new things were changing. In fact, things had been changing for a couple of weeks. Emily, my precious mother, showed new signs that were frustrating. She picked at the dark objects in her food removing anything dark; it was hard to watch the light gradually being pushed out of her life by a permanent darkness. This new darkness was brought on by plaque in the brain that now controlled her whole being. It made me almost sick to my stomach thinking about the changes taking place in her brain. The sparkle in her eyes was also changing, her mood was changing, mom was rambling at night, but nothing seemed to settle her except long rides.

Mother also complained in the evenings with headaches, her throat hurt or she was tired. Sometimes she had ear aches and I would put Sweet Oil in her ears, which relieved her immediately. Emily, my precious mother, was beginning to go through the dark side of dementia, the dark tunnel where there would gradually be no more light. The blunt awful, horrendous, tragic news, confirmed by the MRI, was diagnosed as Alzheimer's. I felt such pain when I heard the awful news! She had been my child for almost eight years, but now my mind raced through thoughts of what would be next. Yes, she had slapped me, spit in my face, pinched me, bit me and tried to kick me many times. I knew this was not like my mother. How do you prepare for the ultimate, knowing we all have to face something in our life, but I had cared for mother since 2000? She had become bonded to my hip joint. She was with me seven days a week. I had given up all my life, except working, to care for her. What would become of her? My mind raced through so many thoughts. "Oh dear Lord," I thought, "Please don't force me to put her into a nursing home." I began googling and searching again for answers. It would be a moment by moment, day by day; week by week not knowing what would be next.

Alzheimer's disease was not pleasant. I had raised four children, watched them grow, experienced the teenage years, but to start all over with an adult going through phases of much the same gave me chills of fear. Could I handle this child? What would she do next? Where did she hide her treasured belongings? How could she relive the past and feel her mother so close, think Frank was in the next room, wonder why Johnny had not come home, why Woodrow had taken so long to go up to Sam's or why did Murphy take so long to come home. She sometimes thought her children were in bed with her and wondered through the house trying to find them explaining they were just playing tricks on her. It became a daily routine to hear her go through reliving the loss of each member of her family. She talked to the TV like the people were with her, but I could tell there was a new shadow spreading over her, one that was engulfing her very life and inch by inch, day by day, minute by minute, it was taking mother into a dark side of life. One that I did not want her to go to, but I knew there was nothing I could do, but to continue my loving care for her.

It was with sorrow to painfully tell her they had all gone to heaven. Their spirits were wondering through Kits Cemetery or Resthaven Cemetery, but she cried and went through the same heartache each time I had to break the awful sad news how we were all that was left of the family. "Mother, we still have Shirley and Kim next door," but it would be the same deep agonizing look in those beautiful hazel eyes. I hated for the sun to start going down. Sun downing – I had heard this phrase and now understood the meaning of what it actually meant the changes taking place in her twisted mind. The agony was the same each time. "But, I just saw mother pass by the door," she persuaded. "She will be right back!" At night when I tucked her to bed she would say, "Frank will be coming to bed shortly." I would gently sit on her bed, rub her sweet face, brush her hair back and tell her that Frank was in heaven with the rest of our family. The strained hurt nearly broke my heart as I went through the same ordeal every day. I knew the signs, watched her face, listened to her voice, but it would be me to break the same sad news every day. They were all gone. How do you explain the loss of fifteen siblings, parents, two husbands and two children to someone that relives every day thinking they were still alive!

I had a numb feeling, mostly scared, because I was so afraid that one day I would have to put mother in a nursing home, the place I promised she would never go. Could I always care for her? The signs of losing control of her were real. Thank God for Phyllis. I leaned on her for support and she understood mother's feelings. She loved mother dearly and assured me that she would always be there when I needed her. And Kim was next door and a great support.

Life is strange. The savagery of disease, cancer, Alzheimer's, heart, diabetes or a tragic end is all the same. How do you face the end? I can tell you how I faced it as I remember it. When mother often repeated the same things over and over, I had to remember when I was growing up and she had such patience with us, showing us how to tie our shoes over and over, reading the same stories over and over. When she did not want to bathe, I had to remember crying and telling her I was too tired from playing and did not want a bath over and over, but her patience with me was unending. She assured me I would feel better after my bath. When she had problems trying to find the words she wanted to say, I remembered when she helped me choose the words when I could not think of just the right word I wanted to say. When she did not understand how to use the microwave, I remember when we got our first electric stove and she had to teach us how to use the burners and the oven over and over. I remember trying to make sugar toast in the oven when we did not have a toaster and she would gently explain to use the broiler part of the stove and not the lower oven, even though many times I burned the toast. She never got angry, but was very patient. When I could not remember something she had told me, she did not say, "I told you already," instead she told me again. I knew I had to have patience when she could no longer remember things. I never told her I had already told her and was tolerant of her as she had been with me.

When mother began to get slower, I did not push her to hurry, instead I remembered when my legs were short and I could not keep up with hers, but she would slow down, hold my hand and take her time with me. She was now my little girl and I wanted to be the best mother I could possibly be to her. I treated her with love, kindness, respect and patience.

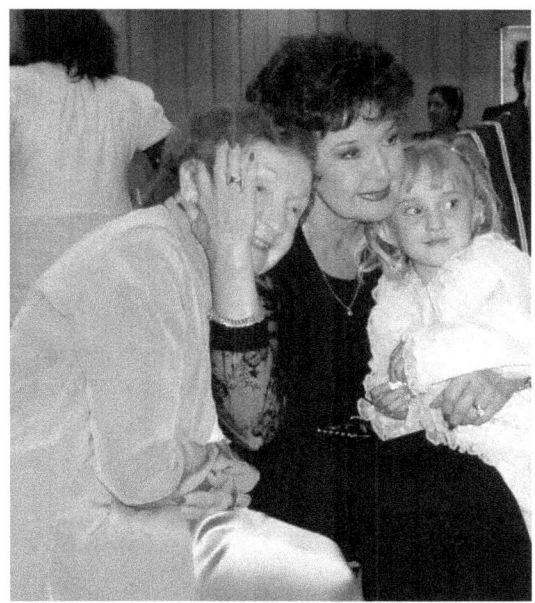

Mother, Joyce, and Bailee

Saturday's were repetitious. Mother watched for Phyllis while I prepared her breakfast. She first went to the front porch, stood watching every car that passed, comes to the kitchen and comments about the fat person walking, and wondering why Phyllis had not arrived. Emily never forgot those closest to her heart. She loved Phyllis, but she forgot that she did not come on Saturdays. She understands that I worked very hard. She was still extremely observant and never missed an opportunity to say, "Honey, you are so pretty." God, I think, this lady was amazing! She happened to be my mother and a very special lady. She had survived so many tragedies and found a way to get through them all without losing it. Her education never went beyond the 6th grade, but her knowledge was that of a PhD! I learned early that common sense takes you through life, forces you to solve problems, but a formal education will land you the job you wanted. Mother already had landed the job she had wanted many years ago when she first laid eyes on daddy and he saw her playing on the swings at the school yard. She talked about how much he looked like Clark Gable, but she would tell you quick that her Calvin was much better looking than Clark Gable. It was her job of a lifetime of caring. I had ached to know what mother's IQ could have been. She calculated, thought out a problem, found a solution and mastered the impossible. You could almost hear the wheels turning as she worked on a project. She was meticulous and pushed herself for perfection. Our little house on Sookie Ridge was immaculate and I could still see the same qualities in her as she walked through the house making sure "everything" was in place.

Finding something strange meant losing it to her bedroom in a secure place, a drawer, hanging in her closet or tucked under "pillow." Everything was neat. In fact, you might have called mother a "neat freak," but that was my mother. She taught me to always keep everything organized and in order, to make my bed the minute my feet hit the floor and do dishes the minute everyone finished. "Don't put off tomorrow what you can do today," she would say. Her glass of milk had to be placed "just so," or the napkin folded to a "perfect" square. She still matched her clothes although often she dressed summer when it was winter or Christmas when it was the 4th of July. It was just before Christmas when she came walking out of her bedroom one morning wearing a beautiful pair of sky blue pants, a pastel yellow summer sweater and a pair of long green and white beads. I teased that she looked like St. Patrick's Day and she laughed 'til she nearly cried. She was a bundle of laughter and pure joy. You could see the twinkle in her eyes, just like her father's, my grandfather, as she told stories that were funny. Of course the stories got mixed up, twisted, blown up, but they were always the same with the laughter. Everyone enjoyed her stories and laughed when the words were repeated over and over, but a little different each time they were told. "I love your mother and her stories," Phyllis had said so many times. "She keeps me and Ann buckling with laughter. She is so quick and never misses a trick. Oh, you have to watch her closely if you take her in a store because she loves anything that sparkles." I often reminded Phyllis she was allowed one phone call and she would remind me that her son was on the police force. There were many times I could not return an item not knowing where it came from.

Mother loved children and animals and the new cat, Shadow, that Kim found dropped at the office turned out to be her best friend. Shadow watched every morning for mom to come to the back door to feed her. She sat on the railing to the back door and leaned over peeping in the window watching anxiously for mother. The minute the door opened she followed mother to her food bowl and mom would stoop gently caressing her as she ate. They made a wonderful bond and every morning mother got up she would ask about Shadow. This amazed me when she could not remember simple things like where the bathroom was, or the refrigerator, but she remembered Phyllis and Shadow. I would give her a cupful of cat food to feed Shadow every morning. This cat sat at the back door on the hand rail and waited for mother knowing she would be there. It was like they needed each other. Sometimes I found the cup in the refrigerator, or in the living room, but she could remembered Shadow needed food even if she could not remember where the cup belonged after feeding her. When Shadow went into heat I immediately asked Kim to take her to the vet. This cat was more like human than animal.

The day Kim brought her back home was the day she moved inside the house. It started with just a small litter box in my office with food and water. Then she showed signs of not scratching on the furniture, so she graduated to the great room on the sofa. I knew I had the perfect baby sitter while I did other things throughout the house. Mother would sit for long periods of time on that sofa with Shadow and Shadow never missed a moment to make sure mother's hands were touching her. Yes, these two made a perfect team and Shadow became my baby sitter.

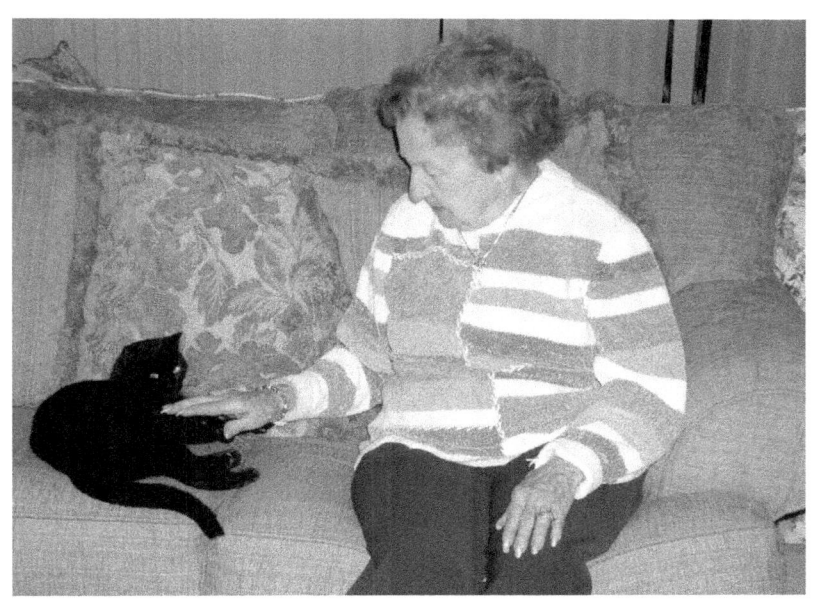

Shadow and Emily – December 7, 2007

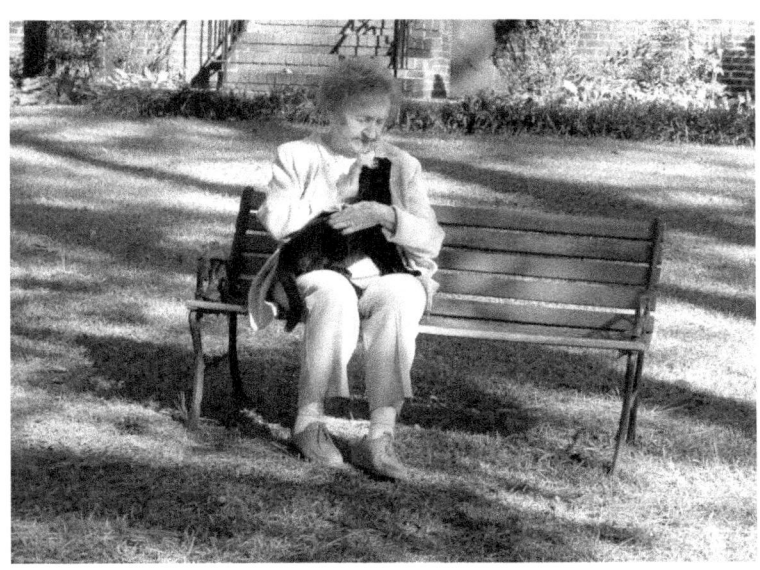

I remembered reading a story about Ike Eisenhower. Ike admired his mother and he told the story about playing games as a child. He was very competitive. One time his mother had made homemade cards. He said she was very religious and they would not buy the real cards. One night they sat at the table and played a simple card game. When the cards were dealt, Ike knew he had a hand that was impossible to win and began complaining. His mother suddenly stopped the game and said, "Boys, put your cards face down on the table. Ike, this is meant toward you because you are complaining. In life, we are often dealt hands we do not want, but we have to deal with the hands we are dealt." Ike knew what his mother meant and he also knew his mother was a woman of wisdom. Mother was also a woman of wisdom, plus she always dealt with her cards as they came. Now I see her trying to still deal, but things have made drastic changes for her that she had no choice in having to deal with.

Mother was small in her frame, 4' 11" in her time, but age had taken its toll on her size. I admired her spunk. It had taken me years to understand her, but now, she was my child and in my care. I found myself playing mind games with her to get her to respond. Sometimes it worked, sometimes it did not. I could see the reflection of her thoughts coming and going. Here one minute, gone the next. I could give her a candy bar and turn her around, the moment would be gone. I knew her span of attention was gone forever. Sad, yes, but she continued to be a highlight in my life.

CHAPTER 22 - A Christmas to Remember

It had been almost eight years since mother left Kentucky to make her home in Alabama. The years had flown and mother seemed to stay the same. She still weighed 119 lbs stark raving naked, she still picked anything unusual out of her food, and she still liked pretty clothes, flashy jewelry and chewed her food forever. I cannot see a lot of difference in her except she is slower and the memory is worse. She no longer reads or worked her crossword puzzle books, but she does enjoy the World's Funniest Videos or watches CNN. She has always enjoyed the news of the world. She had a thing about fat people and never missed an opportunity to comment about how they should lose weight. It was often embarrassing, but it was also a hot subject for her.

Christmas was a few days away and I began talking about what fun this year would be. We had enjoyed having Aunt Ruth, Uncle Harold, Judy and her mother, Jeffrey and his new bride Emily,

Jamie, Calon, Kim, Jeromy and Christie for Thanksgiving. What a fun day that had been and mother especially enjoyed Emily because she had the same name.

Jeromy and Kim put up our tree and things were getting exciting. Mother loved gifts, but she never bothered gifts under the tree. Strange she would take other things and "tuck" away in her room, but she left the gifts alone. I constantly held my breath thinking something would come up missing. Like Thanksgiving, when Kim found the new box of Russell Stover's Chocolates under the sofa pillow in the formal living room. And my new silk pajamas were folded in my office desk drawer. She always made sure there was a "place" for everything and everything in its place – lol

This 2008 Christmas was especially the most rewarding of all our years. My sweet son, Chuck, and his family came Christmas Eve and we enjoyed a large breakfast with all my children and grandchildren. Mother was the main focus and we took lots of pictures making this a special day having four generations together. I remembered the previous year thinking she may not be with us another year, but here at 90 she was going strong as ever. It was one of the happiest moments of my life having everyone together. Kim had moved from Florida, then Jeromy followed, Chuck was living in Birmingham with his wife Beverly and their sons, Holden and Landon. Christie, Kim's daughter was also living here in Jasper. As we held a circle of hands, I felt God had leaned down and kissed me with His blessings. It was definitely a day of thanks.

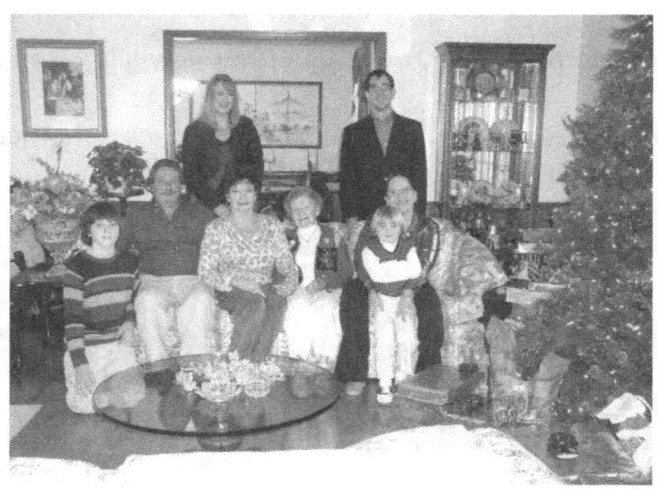

Holden, Chuck, Joyce, Mother, Kim Landon, Bev and Jeromy standing

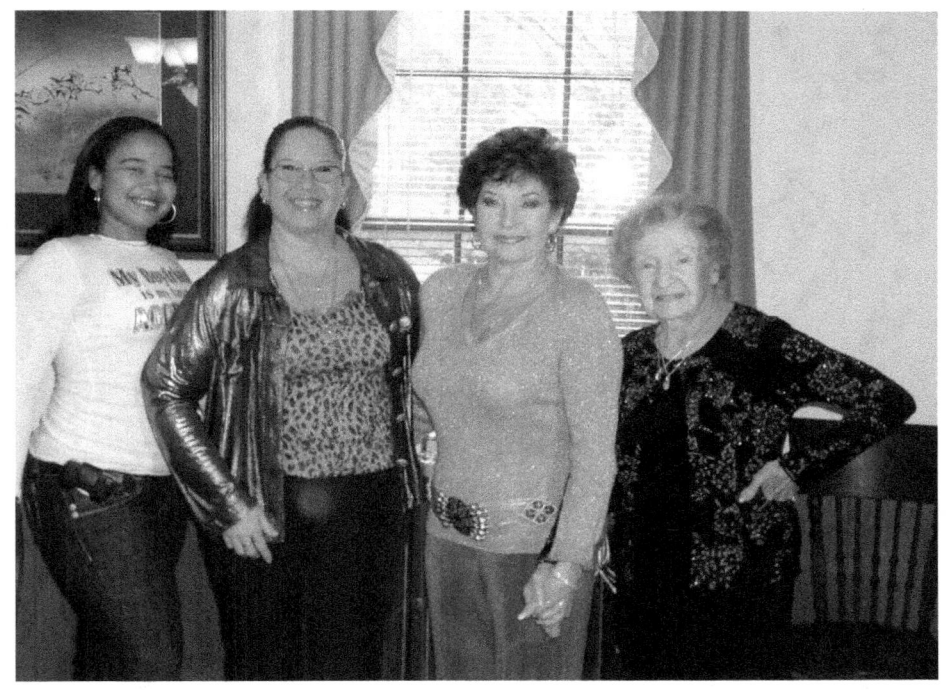

Christie, Kim, Joyce, Mother

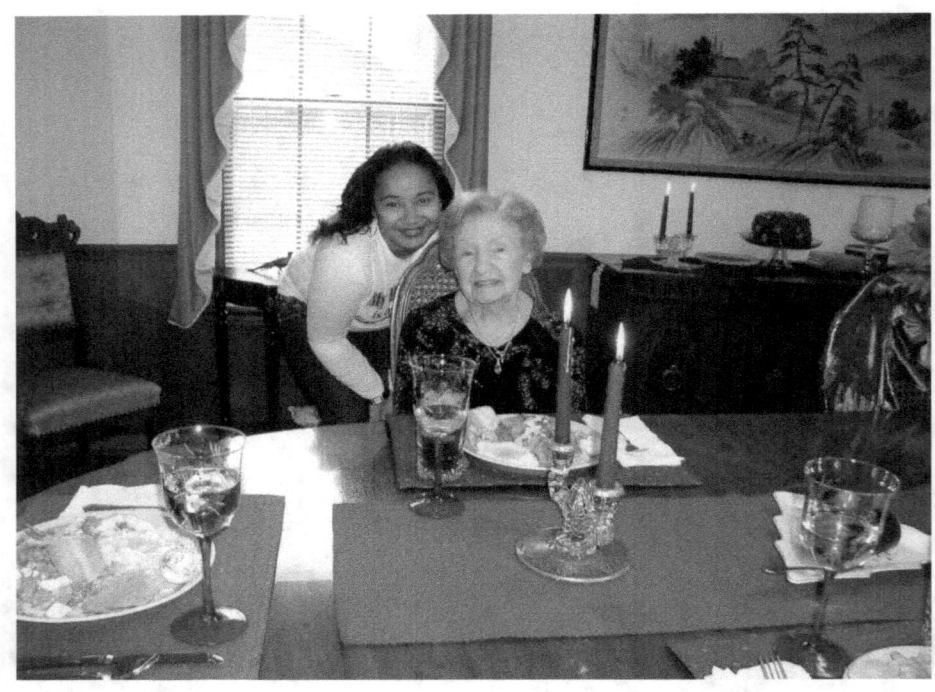

Everyone laughed as mother put cranberry sauce on her mashed potatoes. She loved sweets. Phyllis shared the secret for getting mother to eat chili by putting a pack of Sweet n' Low on it. In fact, she added Sweet n' Low to her salad, and other foods. It made me wonder how many old people starved from not enjoying their foods. My mother was definitely surrounded by lots of love and everyone noticed if she lost her appetite. Phyllis always found a way to get mother to eat and it was through this little packet of Sweet n' Low that made the difference with eating or not eating. I have watched her dip cornbread into ketchup laced with Sweet n'

Low. It almost makes one gag to watch these things, but I often

have to remember that I too woild be there one day – will you?

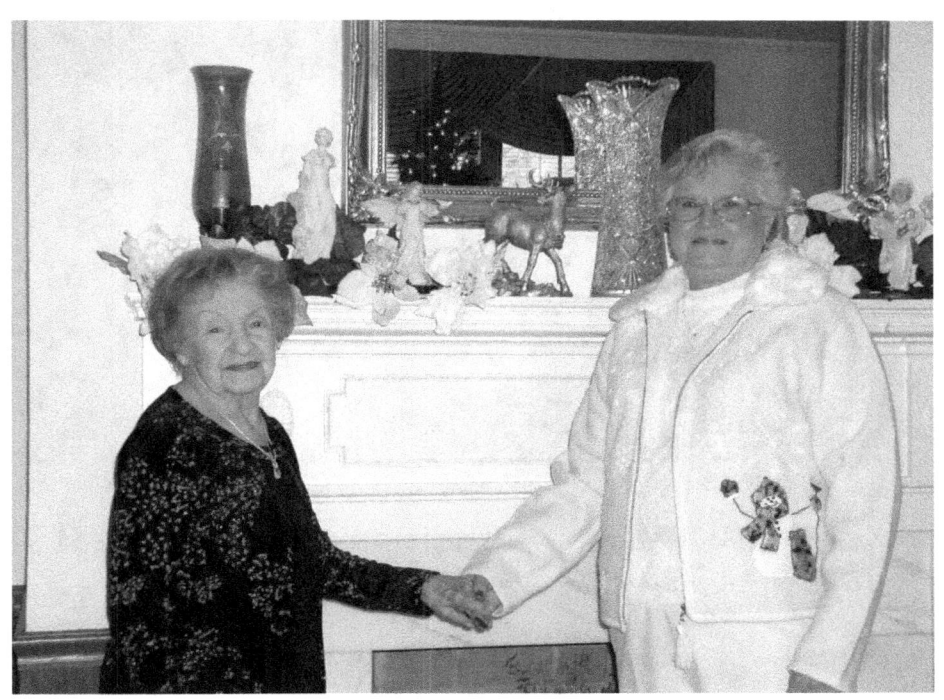

Buddies – Mother and Phyllis (Christmas 2008)

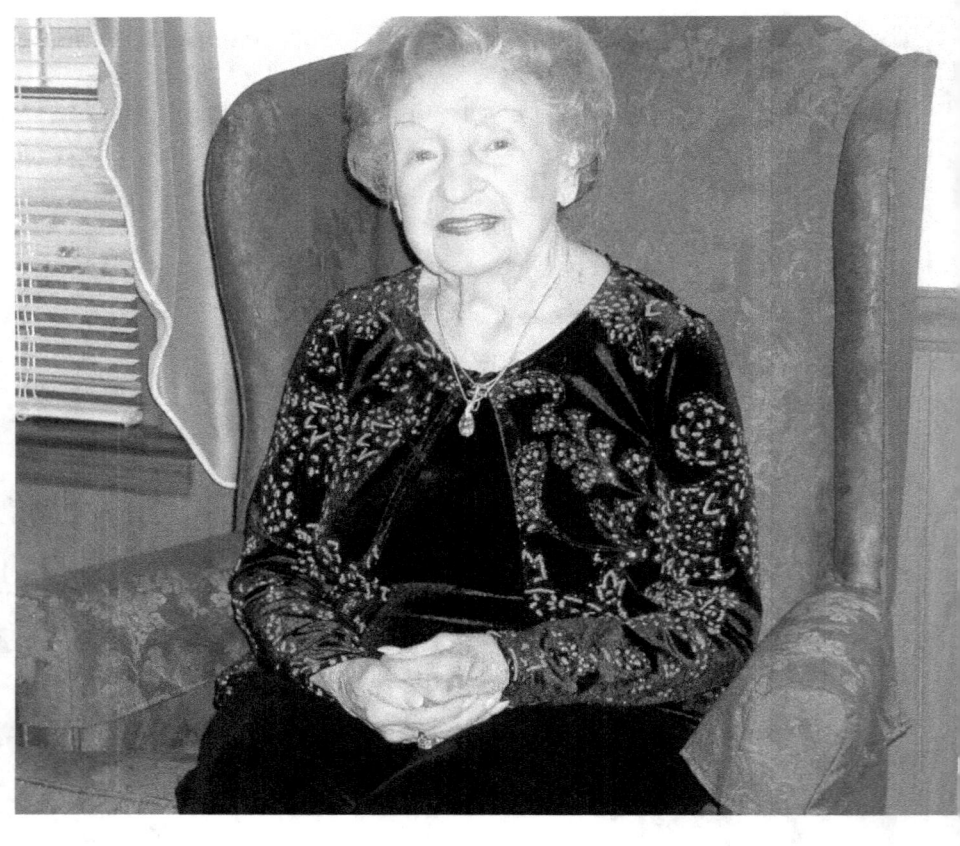

Mother – A Very Special Lady – 90 years old – I kept her looking like a million dollars

CHAPTER 23- The Rhinestone Necklace

Shadow was the newest addition to the family. She actually acted like a human making herself right at home. Mother loved Shadow's attention. Shadow loved mother's attention. They were definitely bonded.

I had this funny feeling about Shadows new pink Rhinestone collar. Mother mentioned how pretty it was, but nothing seemed to be out of the ordinary until the morning mother let Shadow out of the house. I was upset and worried the male cats would kill her. When I told mother she could not let Shadow out, she got mad with me. I said, "Mother, Shadow will get killed if you let her outside." She said, "Joyce Ann," a name she used when she was mad, "I did not let Shadow outside." I continued that it was no one else because no one else was in the house. She continued arguing with me and finally said, "Why I would not do that to Shadow. I love that cat so much I even gave her one of my best necklaces!" With that I could not hold it back. It was so funny. I had just said the night before to Kim that I hoped mom would not take the Rhinestone collar off her neck. I said, "Mom that is a Rhinestone collar, not a necklace." She said, "Joyce Ann, don't you think I know the difference between a rhinestone collar and one of my best necklaces." The next night Shadow jumped on the sofa and mother gave her lots of special attention. I left the room for no more than five minutes, and then suggested it was time for bed. When I started helping mother undress, I noticed a large bulge in her right pocket. I said, "Mother, what do you have in your pocket?" She said, "Oh, nothing, just a few things." When I had her empty her pockets in my hand – lol – there was Shadows Rhinestone collar! I said, "Mother that is Shadow's Rhinestone collar." She said, "Why it is not, that is one of my best necklaces. Shadow can't wear my necklaces." With that I slipped it on my arm, tucked her to bed and left the room. Days are full of surprises and mysteries!

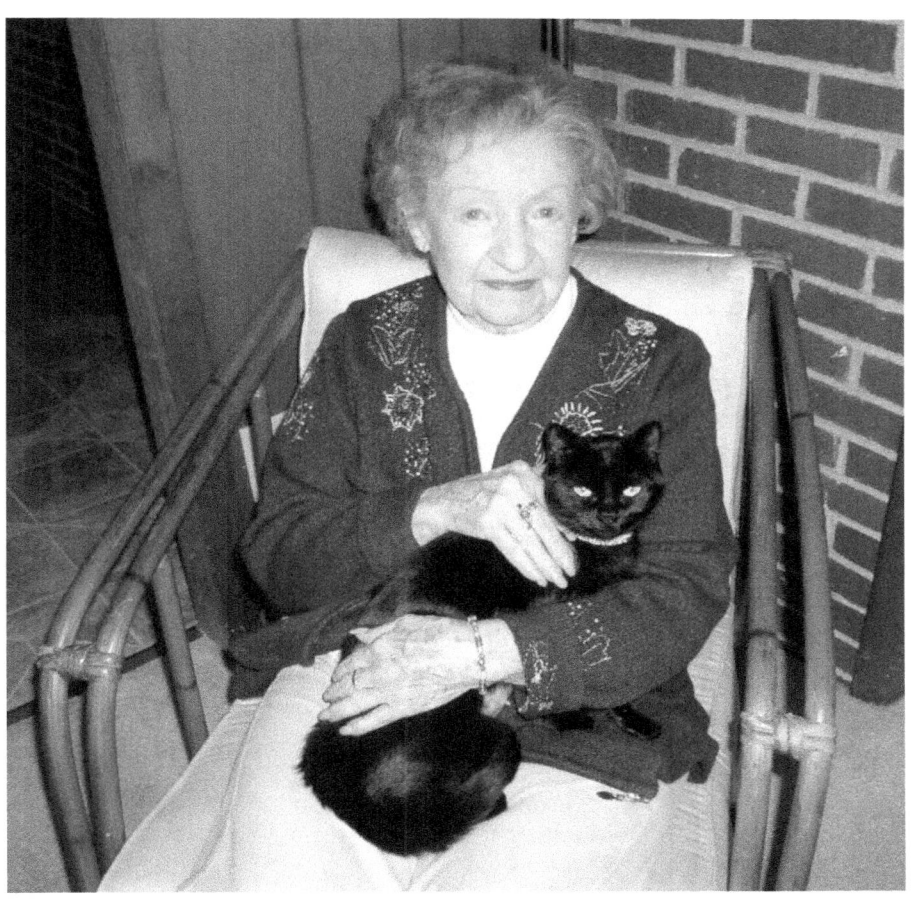

Shadow with the Rhinestone collar

CHAPTER 24 - The Caregiver's and Bumpy Boobs

Phyllis began, "I can see her getting angry and then she starts to get nervous, so I just change the subject and she forgets in a second." We laughed and I said, "I do the same thing!" We stood in the kitchen talking about how we kept her from getting upset. We both loved my mother dearly. She was a handful at times. Phyllis had been around for more than six years now. She knew mom's habits, what made her angry, what she enjoyed, and what she loved to eat. Phyllis continued, "I can tell when something bothers her. She will tell you in a heartbeat that this is her house, she cleans it every day and cooked dinner." We laughed together.

I continued, "I know not to have a serviceman come while she is here. She gets mad and tells them to get out of her house. That she did not order that or it was fixed or no one wants what they have." Mom was a tough lady and continued at her age to fight for her rights. She stood her ground. I bought a beautiful lounge chair, with all the comforts of heat, vibrating and tilting. The thing was so heavy I could hardly move it. I kept finding the chair moved forward in the great room and worked hard to get it moved back. I honestly thought the vibration of the chair was rocking it forward until I realized it was mother moving it.

One morning I told Phyllis the chair was in a strange place, and it was disconnected. She said, "Well, Joyce, I walked in yesterday and hardly turned my back and found the chair all the way back against the wall." I said, "Mother obviously moved it!" We could not understand how she could have moved that chair, because it was very heavy. It was something daily with mother, but we both accepted her as she was.

Mother had a slight cold so Phyllis took her to the doctor just for observation. That night I tucked mom to bed and she complained with a pain in her rib cage. I worried about pneumonia at her age, but not thinking I let it pass and hoped it would be okay. A couple of days later, after Phyllis and I had talked about the chair, it hit me. Mother had moved the chair and pulled something in her ribs and I could not wait to tell Phyllis. When she moved the chair she had strained herself and caused pain in her chest.

Reva began coming on Friday's to care for mom and Phyllis could now have three days off. I often let Reva also come on the weekends sometimes to give me a break. Mom's mood swings were progressing. I could see big changes coming. I was lucky she slept through the nights. She rarely got up for bathroom duties because I now used the adult panties. I now had to completely change everything and it took me extra time before I left for work. The sitters always took mom out for lunch on Fridays and I made sure she looked like a million dollars! Her hair was in place, her makeup perfect and I dressed her like a princess.

The sitter would come, prepare breakfast and sit with mother. Mother loved eating, so this was her favorite meal, giving me the opportunity to slip out the door. The laundry and house were always in order before I left making sure the sitter had nothing to do except keep a "watchful" eye on my mother. It was very difficult to keep up with someone who was slick as a lizard and sly as a fox. Mother would pretend to go to the bathroom, but instead she would be rearranging rooms, all the rooms, placing clothes in my office drawers, spoons in her nightgown drawer, sneaking in my room to change out my clothes or plundering through drawers. It was amazing to find strange things in strange places. She was like a "bad" child that would not listen. When she looked really serious, I knew she had something up her sleeve. When she had a twinkle in her eye, I knew she was good. I could tell in a heartbeat if she had or had not done something – and of course, she could never tell you what she had done as it had already quickly escaped into some distance part of her tiny brain, a brain that could not function, a brain that kept you guessing, a brain that was all messed up and twisted. It was a continual guessing game. Did she, or didn't she. Where was she, what was she doing now?

Jewelry was her big pleasure or anything that was shiny. One day I noticed one of the rings she was wearing had a stone missing. I suggested changing it to get it fixed. Months prior she had been wearing a special ring I bought her with 14k gold, but only Zirconia's, was missing from her finger. "Why worry," I thought, "she has lost the ring and put it out of my mind." Within days after I took the ring with the missing stone off her finger, the original ring appeared on her finger. Sometimes you feel you are losing it and wonder if you are seeing things. It also makes you feel someone is playing dirty tricks on you, but mother honestly did not realize what she was doing.

Mother's humor was contagious. One night I was helping her change into her pajamas, picked up a hanger and hung the pants on the hanger several times in a row. The pants kept falling to the floor and she stood there watching me and screamed with laughter clapping her hands together. I got so tickled watching her and finally realized the hanger was broken. The hanger looked okay when I hung the pants on, but when I would turn lose to put back in the closet they just fell to the floor. She stood there, grabbed her face with her hands and laughed so hard telling me what a funny look I had on my face when the pants fell to the floor. She loved laughing and would enjoy talking and laughing all night. She often begged me to crawl in bed with her and say, "let's talk all night." That particular night we both laughed until we nearly wet our pants. What a woman, what a mother, what a joy.

One Friday evening I came in from work, and found Lois left a note for me on my kitchen counter telling me they would be back soon. When they came in the door, I noticed mother's breasts looking very strange and lumpy. As I talked to Lois, I kept looking at mother's breast until mom finally put her hand on her breast as if to conceal something. In fact, her breast looked bumpy. I paid Lois, fixed mom's dinner, watched a little TV and then took her to get ready for bed. When I pulled her top off, in her bra she had tucked two cookies and several acorns. It was so funny. "No wonder her breast looked bumpy and strange," I thought   I had found eye glasses in her bra, spoons and forks in her bra, but this definitely was a first with cookies and acorns in her bra. They were green acorns and I wondered where she had picked them up, but I would definitely have to ask Lois. I pondered as I continued getting her ready for bed.

I always loved watching mother's face. It was a dead giveaway to what this little lady was thinking. She always had such an innocent look on her face, one that would melt you, but when she was up to something she had this sort of twinkle in her eyes and she would kind of hold her mouth, just so to one side, and I knew the wheels were turning again.

Dementia is a disease that is very complicated as it can progresses very quickly, or very slowly. You never know what to believe when they tell you something or if they are making it up. As it progresses, you can tell the difference sometimes, but not all the time. You get to know their mood swings, what makes them angry, what makes them happy, how to change the subject and totally change their mood. They can seem to be rational, but as you talk you realize they are not.

Mother had, at this time, been with me for more than eight years. I had watched her slowly changing, but now I could see the change becoming more rapid, which was scary. The doctor explained she could coast along, as if she was on the surface of a table, and then one day she could just slide off suddenly, as if falling off a table. He explained it could go that quickly and she would not know me or anyone around us. I hoped this would not be true about mother.

At present, she was a funny, little lady that loved to laugh.......sometimes with pointed boobs, sometimes with bump, lumpy boobs and sometimes just boobs without a bra. What a lady – that was my dear, precious, sweet mother.

CHAPTER 25 – Was I going Crazy?

I had just put my eyeglasses on the vanity when suddenly the phone rang. Mother was sitting on the sofa watching TV with a sweet innocent smile waiting for me to return. The call was short just a telemarketer, but the eyeglasses were gone! Now to try to find the eyeglasses, just like finding my clothes in her underwear drawer the day before and the book I was reading suddenly disappeared off my night stand while I was making my bed. She was standing there and in a flash the items were nowhere to be found. First they were gone and then they mysteriously returned. It seemed a ghost was floating among us, maybe through the air, watching my every move and taking my personal things, shoes, purse, hose, bra, earrings, anything that could not be nailed or tacked down. What a nightmare.

Ms Emily, as everyone called her, was a perfectionist. Everything had to be in place. The napkins folded and placed in just the "right" position, food arranged in order on the plate, pillows on the sofa neatly placed, the chair had to be centered, picture straightened, towels in the bathroom folded just right and hung back on the racks. She had not always been like this, but when her mind began to take on twist and turns in another direction, she also began showing signs of being a perfectionist.

Our house had always been tidy and neat, as she had taken great pride in making a warm, cozy wonderful home. After more than eight years I had learned many of her hiding places. My glasses had to be somewhere close because she was sitting right on the sofa across the room from my chair! She had been so close I could have touched her while I was on the phone. I found it hard to hunt for something when you could hardly see. I asked, "Mom, what did you do with my glasses," and of course was the wrong question to ask someone with this disease. Here one minute, gone the next. The brain cannot function to remember the moments prior and the answer was always the same. "I haven't seen your glasses, Joyce

Ann," she began. I could see the annoyance on her face. I stood there knowing I could not watch the TV programs or read my books without my glasses. "They were right here, Mom," I replied. "I have not seen your glasses, Joyce Ann," she said. That was the name she called me when she really got annoyed. We both began looking for the glasses, but when she stood up, I noticed a strange bulge between her breasts through her sweater – and lifted her sweater. My glasses were stuck in her bra. It was one of the many times she tucked things in her bra. I knew one day I would look back, read the notes I had made, laugh a little, cry a lot, but going through the states of this twisted disease often left you drained and made you feel you were losing reality.

I had noticed how fragile Mother was getting. She had taken a hard fall the day before but by some strange miracle she was okay. She did drink three gallons of milk a week. Phyllis had taken her for a visit with Ann and they were taking mother for a ride and desert. When mother stepped out the back door of Ann's house into the garage she somehow slipped and went tumbling onto the concrete floor, twisting as she fell and landed on her back. She lay there screaming and crying. Phyllis called me at the office and in the back ground I could hear mother. Ann was already calling 911. I could hear the fear in Phyllis's voice and assured her I would be there and it would be okay. Kimberly, my daughter, would not let me drive. We raced to Ann's house to find mother lying on the concrete floor of the garage. Both Phyllis and Ann were crying, but mom seemed to be okay. I was afraid to lift her and waited for the ambulance. We could hear the ambulance going up and down the highway and knew they were trying to find the house. Ann again called and gave directions. We were relieve when the ambulance finally arrived, took mom to the hospital and everyone was happy to hear she had no broken bones. The doctor contributed her luck to drinking the three gallons of milk weekly. Luckily, she came out okay except for a badly sprained ankle. The next several hours were spent trying to keep her off the foot and putting ice packs on the ankle.

It had been only a few months prior that Phyllis had given me the baby monitor she no longer needed for her grandchild. I remember hooking it up and setting the monitor on high to listen to mother's every move. It was Thursday, October 9, 2008. I pushed my ear to the monitor as I listened to her words to God. "Dear God, you know I love you and I want you to take care of my family. Please watch over mom and dad and Murphy and Dallas, Lord. My family has had such a hard life and please, dear Lord, have mercy on me and my family. Help Bessie and Blanche. You know they never had much money and please dear Lord, take care of them and have mercy on them. Lord, also take care of my sweet brother Woodrow. And also, that boy, Curtis I care for. He is so pitiful and please take good care of them. I love you dear God with all my heart. I pray these things in Jesus name – Dad, is that you out there," she yelled. It was this particular night that I felt humbled by the words I heard from the baby monitor I had placed in her room. I had tucked her into bed and thought she was sleeping, but as I climbed into my own pajamas I had heard the whispers coming through the monitor. It would be a night I would always cherish and remember. The words made me chill to my toes and cry silently in the night as I leaned close and put my ear to the monitor to hear mother's words softly talking to God. I had turned up the monitor not wanting to miss a word and felt humbled as she prayed. I stood there thinking about our past, how she had each of us kneel at the old sofa each night together in family prayer and realized her little mind had been twisted in a sordid sort of way through so many losses and heartache she had, but she still did not lose her closeness with God, His goodness and mercy to her and remembered to always pray for others. She had always been a very humble Christian woman, one that never went to sleep without praying. I knew the disease had not taken away my mother's prayers.

I was closing the drawer to my dresser and she heard me. I went back to her bedroom and asked if she needed anything. She replied that she had heard something, but wanted to know if all the doors were locked. I assured her again that the house was secure, leaned down and kissed her gently on her forehead. She was content. I closed the door telling her goodnight again. That was a night I knew she had escaped back into her past, to be with her family and to think the thoughts she had always thought to never let a night go by without a prayer for others. I realized she felt her father was there in the house with her. She was secure and safe. She had gone back in time, a time before I was born, to the life on the mountains in the little log cabin and drifting off to sleep with the security of her past life. I wondered if I would ever find the girdles, but the twist to mother's mind closed her to the troubles of the world and kept her secure with her loved ones. Yes, Mother was a very special lady and for some reason that night I glanced at my book shelf in my office and my eyes landed on one of her Bibles. She had many Bibles there, and tucked away in the pages of the wonderful book of God she had put many handwritten notes. As I looked at each tiny note with her precious handwriting, I suddenly felt she was near as there among so many other little pieces of paper was one a little piece of torn paper with a scribbled prayer. When my eyes landed on the simple words, I felt humble knowing my mother had a prayer in her heart for others and her family was the most precious gift to her. Tears began to drop from my cheeks as I sat there and read it over and over. I held it in my hands, feeling the paper as if mother was there. I could feel her presence and her warm spirit. I knew in my heart what we had meant to mother, but in her own words she had sat and put it all down on a piece of an old ragged piece of torn paper. I am sure she was meditating when the words came to her. It was so old and faded it was hard to read, but she had kept us close to her heart and close to God. Her three girls were her life. She called us by name from birth, Shirley, Joyce and Carol...

My Prayer for you is deep and strong
It reaches out -
And infolds you long
It whispers Peace
And joy and love.
On God To keep
The ones I love

By Emily

She had been my joy, she had been my love and she had been my

keeper, but I had to reverse that to give back the same she had given to me all my life. I had treated her with respect that we were taught. I valued her for what she had instilled into me. I was tolerant of her during rough times, as she had been with me. I listened when she struggled to try to find the words she so wanted to use. I showed her affection as she had done with me. I found things for her to do to make her feel constructive as she had done for me. I cooked all the foods she loved as she had done for me. I made sure she looked like a princess every day as she had done for me. I was reassuring during times of stress as she had been for me. I gave her privacy as she had given to me. I knew all her feelings were intact and made sure I let her know I understood her. I gave her choices as she had given me. I gave her independency as she had given me. I made sure she did not feel ashamed of anything as she had instilled in me. I met all her needs as she had met mine.

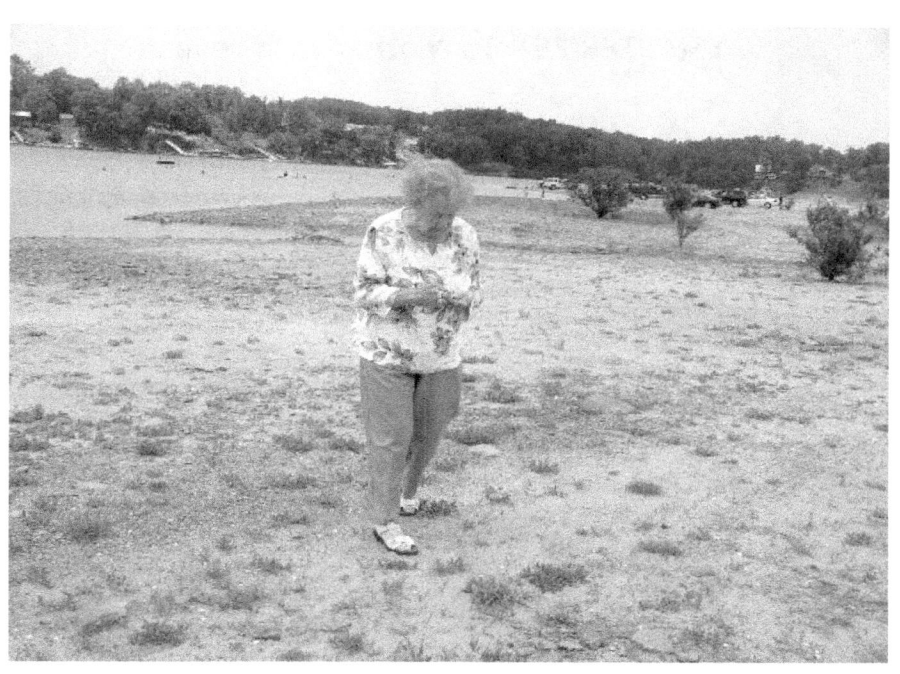

Mother loved finding unusual rocks......birthdays and her grand children .

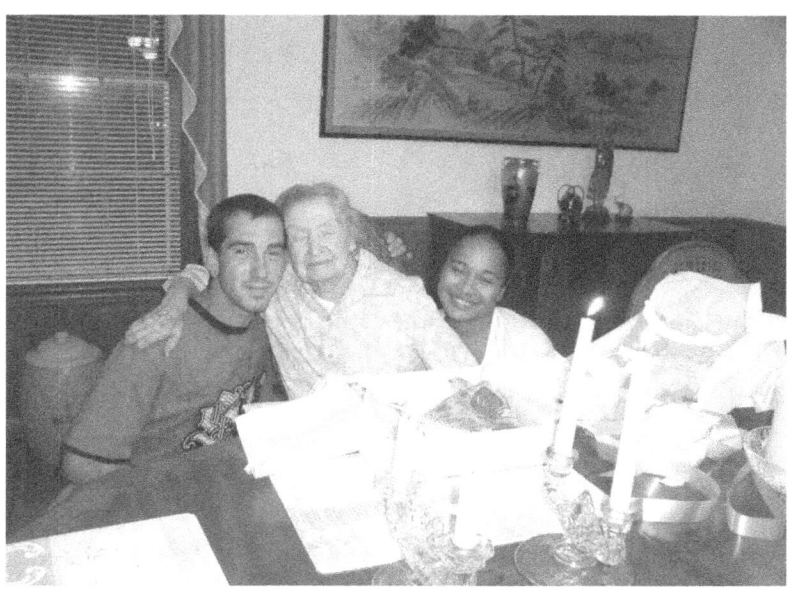

CHAPTER 26 – To Mother with Love

Little did I know it would be mother's last 4th of July, her last birthday turning ninety-two, September 3, 2010, her last Halloween and she would never see the next Thanksgiving or Christmas. It was September 2010 when she fell on the back deck. We had just had milk and cookies, Oreos which were Mother's favorite.

I had been working in the yard blowing the tons of leaves that began to fall and told mother to continue to sit in the swing watching me while I blew the leaves off the rest of the yard. I walked behind my SUV and heard a loud thud, loud enough to be heard above the sound of the blower. When I looked toward the swing mother was not there and when I stepped from behind the SUV I saw her lying on the ground, trying to scream, but there were no words coming out of her mouth. She had a look of panic on her face. We had just been laughing and talking, now she was not able to speak. I began screaming for Kimberly, who lived next door and called 911. When they came they put mother on a board because we knew she had hurt her back and I was horrified she had broken her hip. They carried her to the local hospital where a doctor, specializing in orthopedics, took her to surgery immediately and fused her spine. She had crushed her little spine and was in excruciating pain.

Miraculously mother only spent one night in the hospital and was sent to a local nursing home for twenty-one days of rehab. I went three times daily to visit her, making sure she was dressed properly, eating and had her medicine. The doctor's orders were not to put mother to bed during the day, but to gradually wean her from the wheel chair, encouraging her to walk. He said if he had not done the surgery she would never walk again. I was so proud of her. Here at ninety two she had major surgery, but you would never have known.

I loved taking pictures of mother and took one of her the day we took her to the nursing home for rehab. It would be a horrible day for me to remember. She was very happy in this home, but I still went three times daily to make sure she was cared for, eating right and dressed. It was Friday and I had a long hard week. I had cooked her breakfast that morning and took it to the nursing home, but she was doing so good I told the nurses I would not be back until the next morning; however, at 5:00 pm I decided to go back for fear she would be looking for me.

When I got to the nursing home I noticed a nurse's assistant coming down the hall, but when she looked down the hall suddenly seeing me, she turned and walked back to mother's room, then hurriedly walked to the desk where she proceed to talk to two other nurses. It gave me a strange feeling as I walked by the nurse's station, but getting to mother's room I noticed it was extremely cold and her curtain was pulled around her bed. When I pulled back the curtain I screamed and nearly fainted. This same nurse's assistant had put my mother to bed naked, had put the bed in a downward position with her head lowered as low as it would go and the feet as high as it would go, and the room was ice cold. Mother was clutching a little thin nylon cover with both hands, to her little face with her mouth gapped open trying to scream, but nothing was coming out. She had cried tears that were dry on her face, with still tears coming down. I screamed for the floor manager, but these two nurses and nurses assistant came to the room, one squatting down and showing the one that did this to mother how to adjust the bed. I told her to leave it alone, later wishing I had my camera which was in my purse, but I too was in such shock I could not think straight.

Mother was in a urine soaked bed, even her head was wet with urine and I learned she had been in that position for 7 hours, with no lunch and left in this horrendous position knowing she could not get up. When I hugged mother trying to get her warm, her skin felt like ice. I feared she was going into shock. Her face was bright red from being in a downward position for so many hours and a look on her face that I would never forget as long as I lived.

I later pulled the nurse's assistant aside and asked her why she did that to my mother and she just shrugged her shoulders. I told her I knew she had stripped mother of her clothes, hung them up, put her shoes and socks in the drawer along with her underwear and all she said was, "Yes, I know." I told her that mother was at her mercy and could not understand why she did such a thing. I was furious, but there was nothing I could do. I did call my attorney, but he failed to tell me to take mother to the hospital, where I would have had evidence of the cruel and inhumane treatment they had given her.

Later I learned another family was suing this same nursing home for a similar incident, but for me, it cost my mother her precious life and what a horrible way she had to go. It brought nightmares to me for many months. I also blamed myself for not going back at noon for mother. I also learned this same assistant had asked another nurse why I was so dotting to my mother. She informed me she told her that mother was loved very much and it was sad that other families did not care as much for their mother, so I wondered if she in some sort of sick way did this to see what I would do. I also learned that the nurse's assistants were not supposed to touch the patient, but this particular one got promoted during the remainder of the time mother was there.

Three days after the incident the head nurse kicked mother out of the nursing home saying she was ready to go home and would do much better than to stay the remainder of the twenty one days in the home. They knew mother was dying and did not want her to die in their nursing home. The doctor did not discharge her and I questioned her, but she called for a taxi to take mother home, and ordered a hospital bed for her and forced me to sign her out. There was nothing legal that I could do later. I am stating all this to warn others if they have to put their loved ones in these homes, they must keep a close check on them. Our elderly loved ones are helpless and they continue to lean to us for their good care and security. I felt mother would have lived another ten years had this accident not happened, but the hospice nurse told me she actually died of hypothermia and shock and had lost her mind due to the extreme trauma she had gone through. After that day mother never talked again, she never walked again and she never ate again. What food she had was forced down her.

I remember one night after Kim and I had gotten her into bed, I could hear her little stomach growling. I said, "Mother, are you hungry?" She said, "Uh huh." I now slept in her bed beside her and had the hospital bed put in her bedroom. I got up, got a can of Insure and with a straw I gave it to her. It took two hours to get this bottle of Insure down mother, but I made sure she did not have that hungry feeling. I lay in bed for hours crying and praying for mother, but I knew I was losing her. I could tell by the way she breathed, the struggle she had, and not being able to move herself, not even her arms or her legs. It was such a useless thing to have happened. I would never understand the meaning of what had been done to her, and wondered how this young woman could do such a dreadful, terrible thing.

I did know that mother had left her mark on this little community. Everyone had fallen in love with her and everywhere we went she was known. I loved the way she smiled at others, stopped and talked with a child and petted an animal. Mother was so full of love and tenderness, but it was all taken away at the hands of an uncaring, selfish, mean nursing assistant. I did write letters to the State Board of Nursing and the home was inspected, but they knew this would happen and had prepared for the inspectors that stayed for three days. In talking with an attorney about this incident he told me that they had a huge lawsuit against this particular home, but it would take some years to close it down, but that my mother would have justice one day. Did it make me feel better? No, but at least I felt one day this home would no longer be in business and hoped it would be an example to other homes that cared so little about the elderly.

It was through my visiting niece, Shannon, who was an RN that told me that mother had died of hypothermia and had lost her mind. She also said mother had been put in that position to die. My heart will always continue to hurt every time I think of my mother's strained face and how she could be treated so inhumane when she was such a wonderful, loving, special person.

Mother left my home to be with Jesus November 15, 2010. She was in loving arms and I knew her home would be one that I too would be living in one day. That was some closure to me for what had happened, but I could look back and have so many wonderful memories of my mother. For me, I could not remember bad times. She was always there even when her little mind began to take a turn and twist that began to control her. I could still see her through the clouds of dementia. I could still feel the tender kisses on my cheeks as she sang her Pollywog song, I could still hear the giggle in her voice and at night I could still hear her tip toeing through the house. She no longer had to grasp for the words she was trying to say, she had a new body and I hope one day, that you too can meet my dear, precious, loving, tender, caring mother. Mother always told us that one day she would have a new body, wear a crown of pearls, walk the streets of gold and she would not have to ever worry about growing old. She was no longer my child, she was my angel walking those streets of gold and sitting on my shoulder watching me........I never found the girdles..........

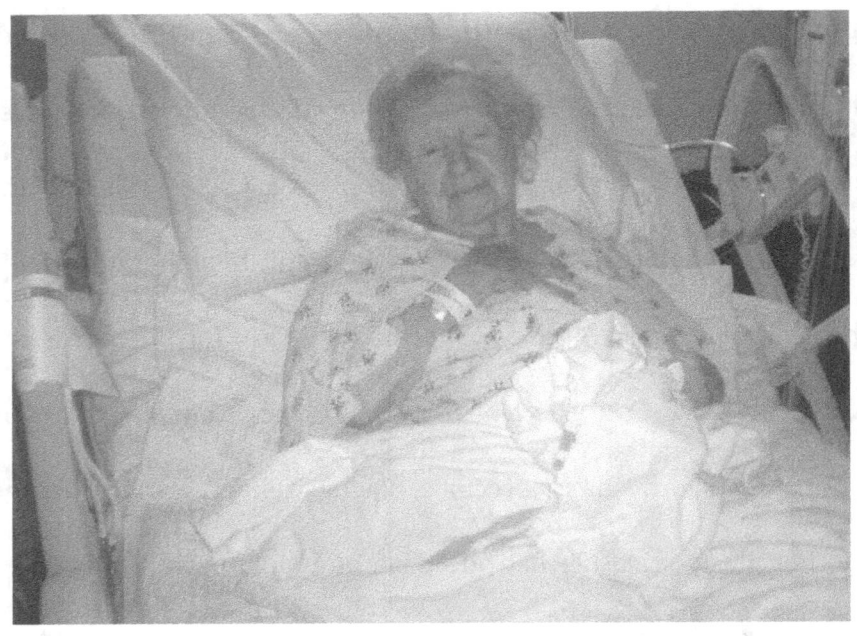

Just after mother coming out of surgery and spending only one night in the hospital, then to rehab for twenty-one days

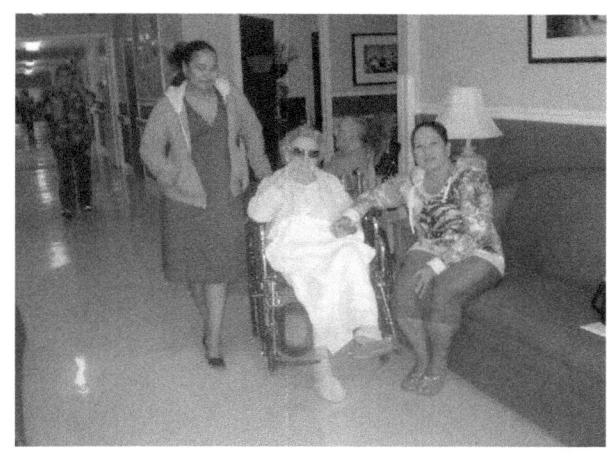

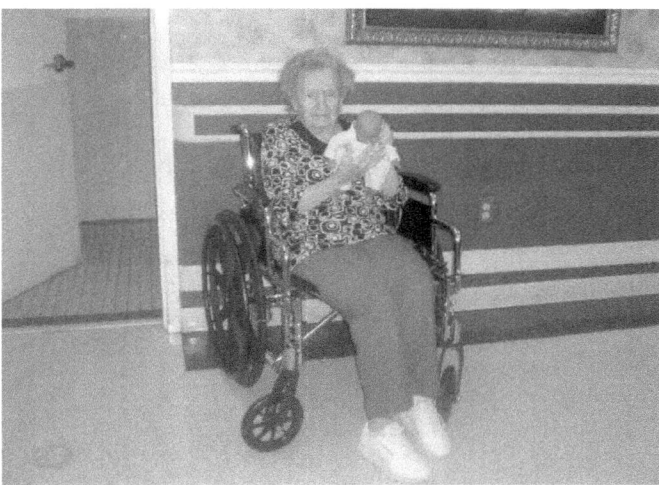

Christie, Mother and Kim and the day before I found her naked in bed.

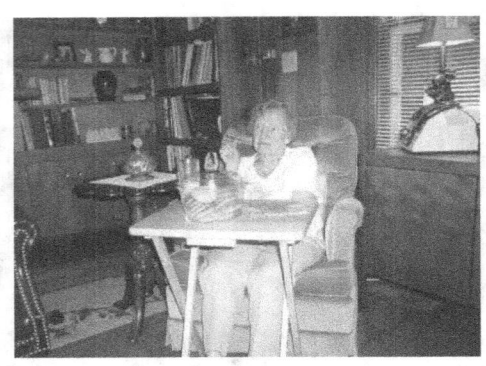

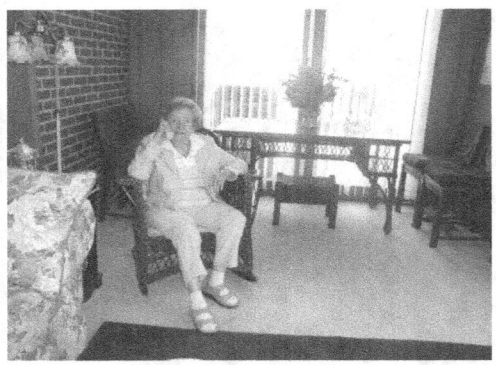

Her favorite chair and eating cookies and milk   and talking on the phone to

Shirley

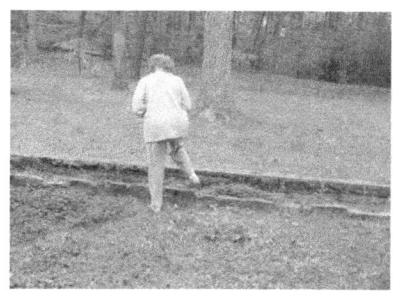
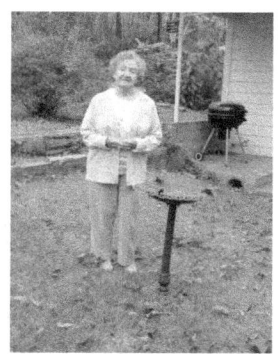

Sneaking off for a visit with the neighbor, an innocent face

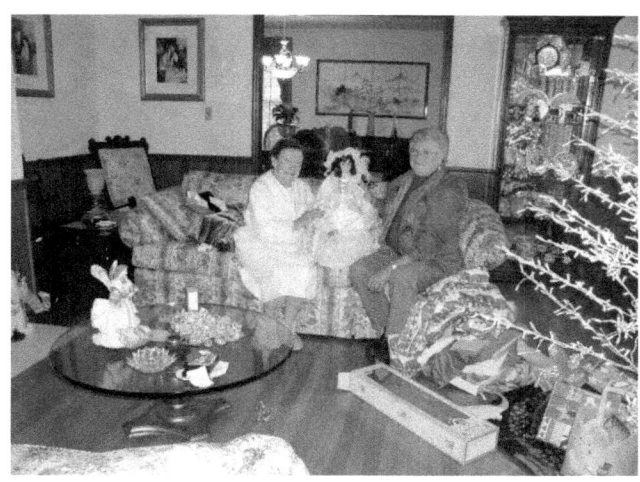

Phyllis gave her this beautiful doll for Christmas 2009

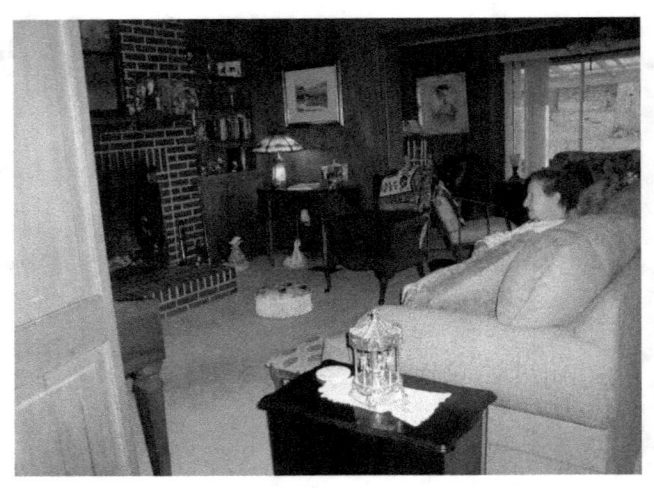

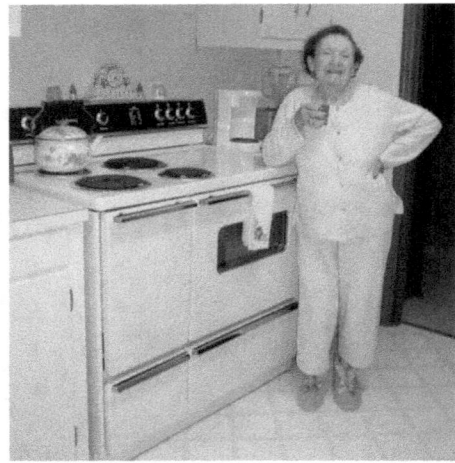

Mother loved watching TV and enjoying a cold glass of milk before bed

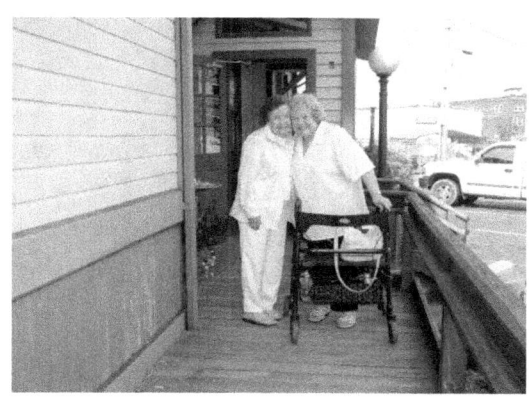

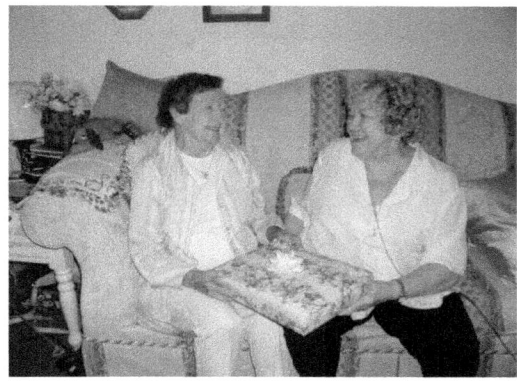

The day we arrived in PA to visit Shirley - exchanging birthday gifts, mother's

Sept. 3rd, Shirley's Sept. 4th

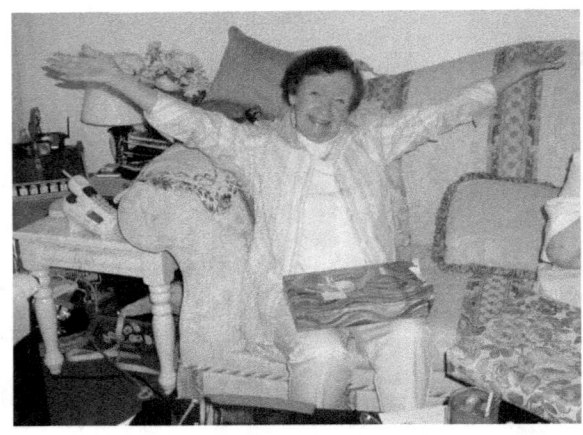

Celebrating their last birthdays, and Shirley in Pennsylvania, 2007

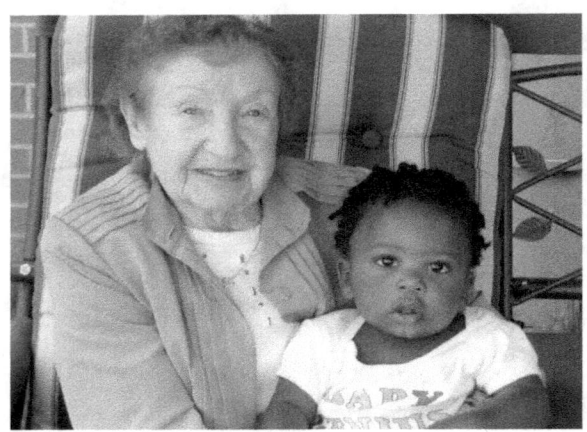

A neighbor's darling baby

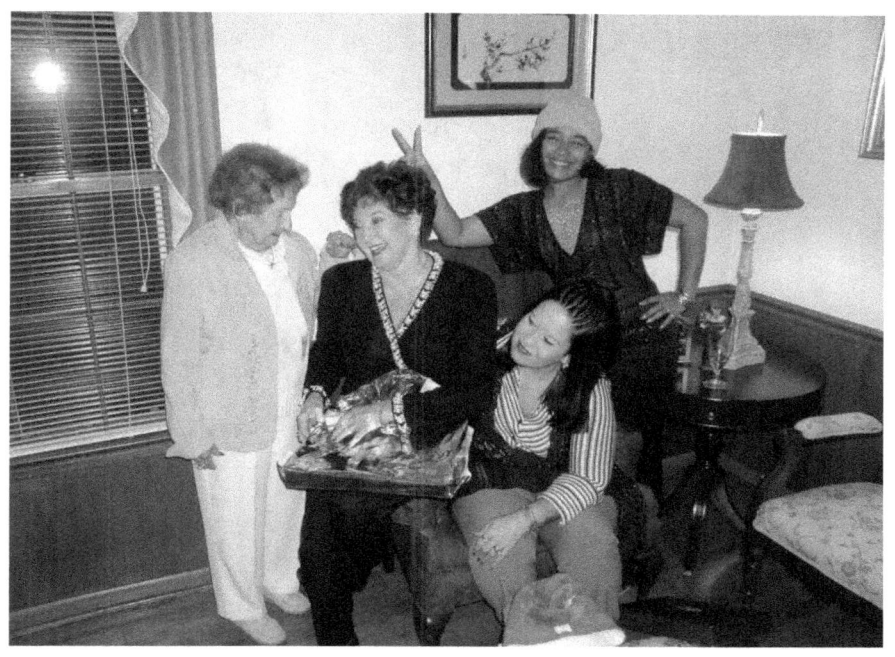

Mother, Joyce, Christie and Kimberly

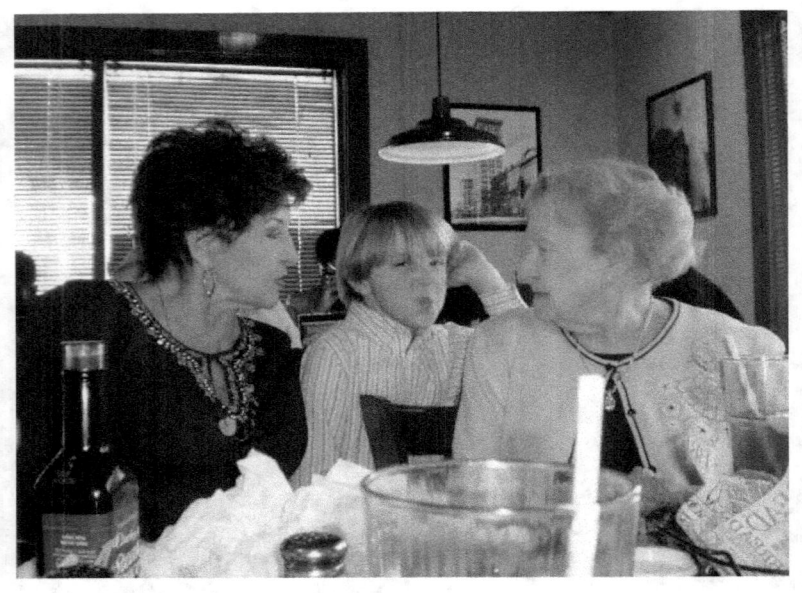

Joyce, Landon, Mother (mother's great grandchild)

Mother loved cookies and milk, talking on the phone, birthday gifts, getting dressed up for Mother's Day, adventures, sneaking off like a child to hunt for things and finding a bird bath that I never knew who owned it, holidays and dolls, walking in the park, eating out with the family, her milk in the mornings, she loved watching TV in the comforts of our home, she loved looking for different rocks always an eye out for an arrowhead, riding in the car on long trips and visiting her daughter, Shirley, she loved animals and children, she loved to laugh and have fun with the family, and she loved her grandchildren. Most of all, I treated mother like she was the same as always, giving her the love and respect that she deserved. I took her everywhere and listened to her stumble for words, but making her feel a part of everything. Mother truly loved living and she was my joy.

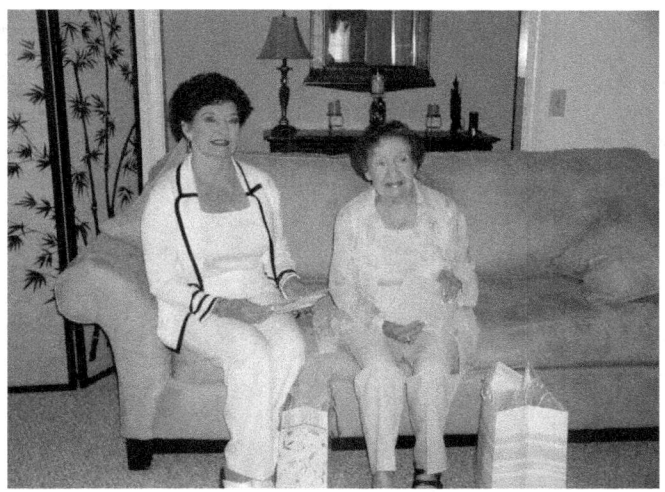

In ordinary life we hardly realize that we receive
a great deal more than we give, and that it is
only with gratitude that life becomes rich.

— Dietrich Bonhoeffer

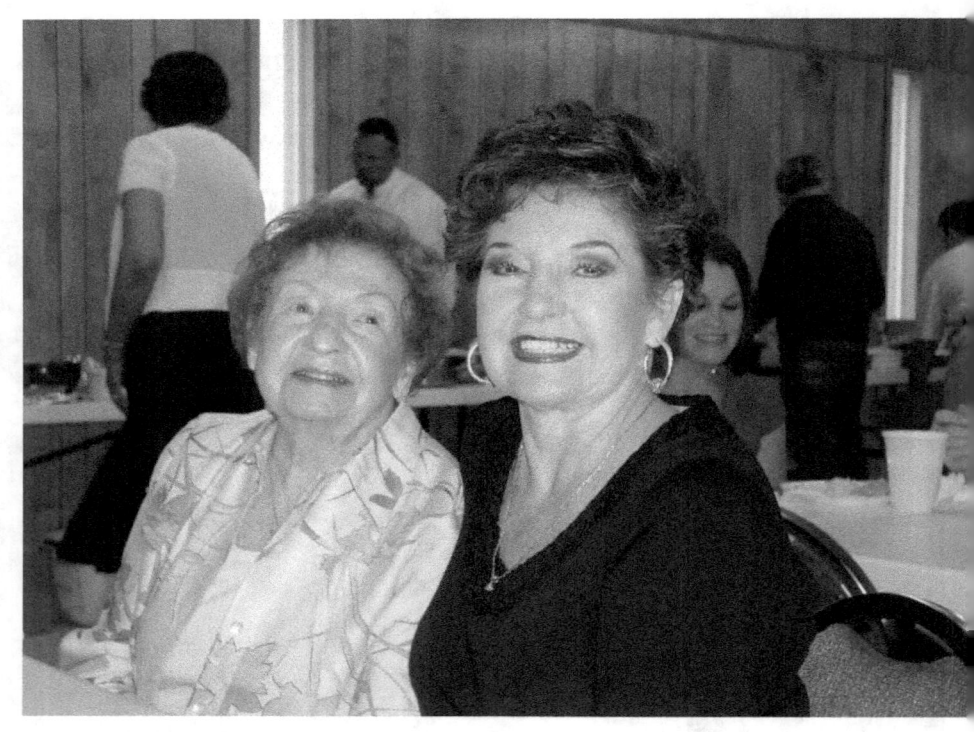

To mother with love, Joyce

I never found the girdles...........

EPILOGUE

Mother was cremated and laid to rest with my daddy in the Resthaven Cemetery, Harlan County, KY next to my sweet sister, Carol. Mother belonged in those mountains. I could never bring myself to visit anyone in that nursing home again.

We were a close family and made sure our loved ones belonged together. I am sure mother is floating among her mother and dad, sisters and brothers, husbands and daughters and I too shall one day join their hands and float among the beautiful mountains we all so dearly loved.

It has been through many friends' stories and blessings that made me write this book. Everywhere I would go someone would tell me something about mother, from her past Sunday school students, to the friends she had made in our little community and also to Ruby, her niece, telling me that mother was the person responsible for her going to church. Mother was loved by everyone she came in contact with and touched the hearts of many and out of this love made me feel I should tell mother's story. About how she also loved everyone and about the real truth in how she was treated in the nursing home rehab. I hope this book will be an eye opener for those who have to resort to these homes for their loved ones and also will help others understand what dementia is all about. You can help prevent tragedies at these nursing homes by being there for your loved ones. I had to be my mother's eyes, hands and protector. Even though I was there for her every day, by missing one single day cost mother her life, but I do know that she is in a better place, a home that she will never have to leave again.